THE COMPLETE IBS RELIEF DIET COOKBOOK

THE COMPLETE IRRITABLE BOWEL SYNDROME DIET GUIDE FOR TOTAL SYMPTOMS RELIEF, BALANCE FIBER INTAKE AND PREVENTING OTHER GASTROINTESTINAL DISORDERS

CATHERINE JONES

Copyright Page

© 2023 Catherine Jones

Table of Contents

Chapter 1: UNDERSTANDING IBS AND DIETARY MANAGEMENT

The large intestine is affected by the common gastrointestinal illness known as Irritable Bowel Syndrome (IBS), which causes a variety of symptoms associated with bowel function. Irritable Bowel Syndrome (IBS) is a functional condition, meaning it disrupts the normal working of the intestines rather than a structural defect in the digestive tract. It is characterized by its chronic nature. This illness is rather widespread and can afflict anyone at any age; however, it is typically found in those younger than 50.

There is likely a complicated interaction of variables that lead to the development of irritable bowel syndrome (IBS), but the specific reason is yet unknown. It is thought that factors such imbalances in gut flora, irregular intestinal muscle contractions, and increased sensitivity to stimuli in the digestive system contribute to the onset of irritable bowel syndrome (IBS). Possible causes of irritable bowel syndrome (IBS) include heredity, mental health issues, and food choices.

Symptoms of irritable bowel syndrome (IBS) can vary greatly from person to person and constitute its defining feature. Gas, bloating, and changes in bowel habits (diarrhoea, constipation, or alternating between the two) are common symptoms. Disruptions to regular tasks and emotional discomfort are two ways these symptoms might lower a person's quality of life.

There is currently no definitive test for irritable bowel syndrome (IBS), hence a diagnosis must be made based on the presence of distinctive symptoms. To make a diagnosis, healthcare providers often look at the patient's medical history, conduct a physical exam, and rule out other possible gastrointestinal problems. Although irritable bowel syndrome (IBS) can not cause colorectal cancer or other major consequences, it is a persistent and unpleasant illness that needs constant attention.

Lifestyle changes, dietary adjustments, and medication are all part of the complex toolbox for managing irritable bowel syndrome (IBS). Finding and avoiding certain foods that may bring on symptoms is a common goal of dietary plans. An integrative strategy for irritable bowel syndrome (IBS) care also places an emphasis on stress reduction, physical activity, and sufficient rest.

The duration and severity of irritable bowel syndrome (IBS) might differ from one individual to the next. Long stretches of symptom remission are possible for some people, while others may have to deal with chronic symptoms all the time. Better focused and effective treatment options for those affected by IBS may become available as research into the underlying causes of this prevalent gastrointestinal condition develops.

Types and Distinction of IBS

Each of the three major forms of irritable bowel syndrome (IBS) is defined by a unique set of symptoms and patterns of bowel movements. In the first kind, known as irritable bowel syndrome with constipation (IBS-C), sufferers report stomach pain in addition to infrequent and firm bowel movements. Stool passing through the colon more slowly is a common symptom of this subtype.

The second kind, irritable bowel syndrome with diarrhea (IBS-D), is characterized by frequent episodes of loose or watery poops. A feeling of incomplete bowel motions and urgency are additional symptoms that may be experienced by those with IBS-D. A shorter amount of time for feces to pass through the colon is commonly associated with this subtype.

In the third kind, known as mixed-type IBS (IBS-M), patients have both diarrhea and constipation simultaneously. Over time, symptoms might change, going from constipation to diarrhea. People with mixed-type irritable bowel syndrome may find it difficult to control their symptoms due to the disorder's variable nature.

Keep in mind that there is still much mystery around irritable bowel syndrome (IBS) and that several variables, such as heredity, intestinal motility, dietary sensitivities, and infection history, may play a role in its onset. It is common practice to exclude other gastrointestinal problems through medical assessments and testing and rely on the presence of particular symptoms when making a diagnosis.

Although there is currently no known cure for irritable bowel syndrome (IBS), treatment focuses on reducing symptoms and enhancing quality of life. Healthcare providers may advise patients to alter their lifestyles, make dietary changes, learn to handle stress, or take medication to alleviate the symptoms of irritable bowel syndrome. Anyone suffering from irritable bowel syndrome (IBS) symptoms should consult a doctor for a proper diagnosis and individualized treatment plan.

Prevalance and What Causes Them

Approximately 10-15% of the global population has symptoms that are consistent with irritable bowel syndrome (IBS), yet this number varies greatly among countries and age groups. The onset of this ailment often occurs in early adulthood, and it is more frequently diagnosed in women than in males.

Irritable bowel syndrome (IBS) is a difficult illness to identify and treat since its causes are complicated and not fully understood. Although there is no one known cause for irritable bowel syndrome (IBS), several variables can bring on or worsen the symptoms. Abnormal gut motility, in which variations in bowel habits are caused by too or underly weak contractions of the intestines' muscles, is thought to be a key component.

When irritable bowel syndrome (IBS) symptoms first appear or worsen, stress and psychological variables are major contributors. Abdominal pain, bloating, and changed bowel habits are symptoms that may manifest in people who are very anxious, depressed, or stressed out. Another risk factor for irritable bowel syndrome is a history of gastrointestinal-related trauma, such as an infection or surgery.

There is evidence that some meals can bring on or exacerbate symptoms of irritable bowel syndrome (IBS) in those who are more vulnerable to this condition. Fruits, vegetables, and dairy products that contain carbs that are not well digested are common culprits. There are certain people who experience gastrointestinal problems because they are intolerant to certain dietary components, such gluten or lactose.

Since there is evidence of a hereditary predisposition for IBS, genetics may contribute to the susceptibility of individuals to the disorder. Having an ancestor who suffers from irritable bowel syndrome increases one's risk of developing the condition, according to the available research. Further research is required to completely understand the genetic basis of IBS, however, because the interaction between genetic components and environmental impacts is complicated.

Millions of individuals all around the globe suffer from IBS. A number of variables contribute to the disorder's etiology, including aberrant gastrointestinal motility, psychosocial variables, food triggers, and a hereditary basis. The development of appropriate management techniques and the improvement of the quality of life for those living with IBS depend on a thorough knowledge of these aspects.

Symptoms of IBS in the Body

Abdominal pain or discomfort is a frequent symptom, and it's usually better after you go to the bathroom. People who suffer from irritable bowel syndrome (IBS) may feel bloated and have cramps every now and then.

Misalignment of the bowel routine is another common sign of irritable bowel syndrome. This can show up as either diarrhea or constipation, or both; in fact, people commonly go back and forth between the two. Discomfort and disruption to everyday life could result from changes in the regularity and consistency of bowel motions.

Feeling full or pressured in the belly, as well as an abundance of gas, are common complaints among those who suffer from irritable bowel syndrome. A lot of people also complain about having to use the toilet more frequently and having flatulence. Worse, the distressing nature of these sensations might amplify preexisting nervousness and tension.

Impacting a person's general health is only one more way that irritable bowel syndrome (IBS) manifests itself. Many people with this disease also report feeling exhausted and unable to sleep, which may be related to the pain and worry they experience. In addition, those who suffer with IBS often find themselves cutting back on social activities because they are anxious about having their symptoms flare up in public places.

Irritable bowel syndrome (IBS) is a long-term health problem; researchers still don't know what causes it, but they do know that factors like food, stress, and intestinal motility might play a role in the onset or worsening of symptoms. In order to get a proper diagnosis of irritable bowel syndrome (IBS) and create a specific care plan to help with symptoms and quality of life, it is essential to consult a medical professional.

Chapter 2: HOW DO YOU KNOW YOU HAVE IBS

A comprehensive medical assessment is necessary to diagnose irritable bowel syndrome (IBS). This evaluation includes taking a full patient history, doing a physical examination, and ruling out other possible explanations of the symptoms. Predominantly, the Rome IV criteria are used to diagnose irritable bowel syndrome (IBS). These criteria state that the patient must have recurrent abdominal pain or discomfort for a minimum of three days per month in the past three months, along with two or more of the following: that the pain or discomfort improves when they defecate, that the pain or discomfort begins when their stool changes in form or frequency, or that both of these things must be present.

First things first in diagnosing irritable bowel syndrome (IBS): get a full medical history that details the symptoms, how often they occur, and how long they have persisted. To be sure there isn't anything more serious going on, a doctor will do a physical checkup and look for any concerning symptoms. Inflammatory bowel disease (IBD), celiac disease, and colorectal cancer are other gastrointestinal conditions that share symptoms; hence, diagnostic testing to rule them out may be suggested. The diagnostic method may involve the use of imaging investigations, such as colonoscopy, as well as blood tests and examinations of feces.

Distinguishing irritable bowel syndrome from other gastrointestinal disorders is a difficulty in making a diagnosis. Inflammation in the digestive system is a hallmark of inflammatory bowel illnesses like Crohn's disease and ulcerative colitis, which may be diagnosed by imaging scans and endoscopic procedures. Celiac disease is an autoimmune ailment that may be detected by blood testing and intestinal biopsies. It is induced by gluten ingestion. In order to rule out cancer, screening procedures such as colonoscopies are necessary, as colorectal cancer might present with symptoms that are similar to irritable bowel syndrome.

It is also vital to differentiate functional dyspepsia and functional abdominal pain syndrome from irritable bowel syndrome. Functional dyspepsia is defined by persistent upper abdominal pain or discomfort, whereas functional abdominal pain syndrome is defined by frequent or continuous stomach pain that does not have a medical explanation.

A thorough medical assessment is necessary for an IBS diagnosis to rule out other possible causes and confirm that symptoms meet the Rome IV criteria. The use of a thorough approach that includes diagnostic testing, patient history, and physical examination helps to differentiate irritable bowel syndrome (IBS) from other gastrointestinal illnesses. This, in turn, allows for a more precise and personalized treatment strategy.

Lifestyle Adaptations on a IBS Diet

If you want to be healthy and live a long time, you need to make certain changes to your lifestyle.

Keeping to a healthy, well-rounded diet is an important consideration. For the best possible physical health, make sure to include a mix of fruits, vegetables, lean meats, and complete grains in your regular meals. Always remember to drink enough of water throughout the day and watch your meal amounts.

Another pillar of a healthy lifestyle is regular physical activity. To improve cardiovascular health, increase muscular strength, and promote flexibility, it's recommended to engage in a mix of cardiovascular activities, strength training, and flexibility exercises. Incorporate muscle-strengthening exercises into your routine at least twice a week, in addition to 150 minutes of moderate-intensity activity or 75 minutes of vigorous-intensity exercise.

A good night's sleep is essential to your health and happiness, yet it's easy to overlook its importance. Get between seven and nine hours of good sleep nightly to help your body and mind recharge. Improve your sleep hygiene by sticking to a regular sleep schedule and developing a soothing pre-bedtime ritual.

Maintaining good mental and physical health requires effective stress management. Make time every day to practice stress-reduction strategies like yoga, deep breathing, or mindfulness meditation. A more harmonious and satisfying existence may be yours when you learn to manage your stress in a healthy way. This can be done through hobbies, time in nature, or spending quality time with loved ones.

An important component of a healthy lifestyle is establishing and sustaining meaningful relationships with others. Build strong bonds with others around you, including loved ones and neighbors. Emotional health and resilience in the face of adversity are both enhanced by having strong social networks to lean on.

In order to promote long-term health, it is crucial to limit the intake of dangerous substances like tobacco and excessive alcohol. Reducing the risk of many chronic illnesses and improving general health can be achieved by quitting smoking and reducing alcohol use.

Maintaining good brain health requires regular mental exercise. Do things that make your brain work, including reading, solving puzzles, or picking up new abilities. Maintaining cognitive function and maybe lowering the risk of age-related cognitive decline can be achieved by continuous mental stimulation.

Leading a healthy lifestyle requires a comprehensive strategy that includes eating well, exercising regularly, getting enough sleep, managing stress, maintaining positive relationships, using substances responsibly, and being mentally stimulated. An individual's quality of life and the future of health and happiness can be improved via the adoption of healthy habits.

Chapter 3: THE IBS DIET

Essential to the management of symptoms related to this prevalent gastrointestinal condition is the Irritable Bowel Syndrome (IBS) diet. A well-planned diet can help individuals with irritable bowel syndrome (IBS) manage their symptoms, which include gas, bloating, and irregular bowel patterns.

The most important thing for people with IBS to do is to figure out what foods set off their symptoms. Common ones include FODMAPs (fermentable oligosaccharides, disaccharides, monosaccharides, and polyols), however they might differ from one individual to the next. Some fruits, vegetables, and grains are high in FODMAPs, which can cause gastrointestinal upset, so it's best to restrict your intake of these foods.

People who suffer from irritable bowel syndrome (IBS) frequently find relief by increasing their consumption of soluble fiber and decreasing their consumption of FODMAPs. Oats, bananas, and other veggies are good sources of soluble fiber. Constipation is a typical symptom of irritable bowel syndrome (IBS), however this fiber can help regulate bowel motions and alleviate it.

Another important aspect of managing IBS is staying hydrated. In order to avoid constipation and keep digestion healthy, it is recommended to drink enough of water. Because they can aggravate gas and bloating, carbonated and caffeinated drinks should be avoided or consumed in moderation.

Yogurt, kefir, and sauerkraut are examples of fermented foods that contain probiotics, which can help those who suffer from irritable bowel syndrome. Live bacteria found in these meals support a balanced gut environment and might perhaps reduce symptoms. To gauge their effect on tolerance, probiotics should be introduced slowly.

People with IBS also need to pay attention to when they eat and how much they eat. One way to lessen the chances of experiencing symptoms is to eat smaller, more frequent meals throughout the day instead of three big meals.

It is critical to record dietary choices and any related symptoms in a food journal while undergoing the irritable bowel syndrome diet. This can be helpful in pinpointing certain causes and directing dietary changes appropriately.

If you want specific recommendations for an IBS diet plan, it's best to go to a doctor or a qualified dietitian. So that IBS may be effectively managed and digestive health can be improved overall, they can give individualized recommendations based on symptoms, preferences, and dietary demands.

Dietary Guidelines for IBS Diet

The precise reason behind irritable bowel syndrome is still a mystery, dietary approaches are vital in alleviating symptoms. Improving the quality of life for those with IBS can be achieved through a tailored strategy that identifies trigger foods and incorporates specific lifestyle adjustments.

The low-FODMAP diet is an important dietary approach for irritable bowel syndrome (IBS). Fermentable carbs that are high in FODMAPs are known to irritate the intestines in certain individuals. Fruits, vegetables, cereals, and dairy products that are rich in FODMAPs should be limited in this diet. The low-FODMAP diet is not a magic bullet; rather, it requires close collaboration between patients, healthcare providers, and certified dietitians to provide the best possible outcomes.

People with irritable bowel syndrome (IBS) are generally advised to increase their consumption of dietary fiber, especially soluble fiber, and to adhere to the low-FODMAP diet. When taken orally, soluble fiber helps ease constipation and other bowel movement irregularities. Oats, psyllium husk, and several veggies and fruits are great places to acquire soluble fiber. To prevent worsening symptoms, it is recommended to gradually incorporate fiber into the diet.

Some people with irritable bowel syndrome may also benefit from taking probiotics, which are good microorganisms that help keep the gut healthy. Yogurt, kefir, sauerkraut, and kimchi are fermented foods that contain probiotics; you may also find them in supplement form. It is recommended to get advice from a healthcare practitioner when determining the most appropriate strains and dose of probiotics, since their efficacy might differ.

An other important part of controlling IBS symptoms is staying hydrated. Those who are suffering from diarrhea as a prominent symptom should drink enough of water to keep their bowels regular and avoid being dehydrated. Because they can lead to dehydration and exacerbate IBS symptoms, alcoholic and caffeinated drinks should be avoided to a minimum.

Eating smaller, more frequent meals and making sure to swallow each bite completely are some mindful eating techniques that might help those with IBS. Keeping a food journal to record symptoms and possible causes can also help in developing a tailored and efficient eating regimen.

Although many people find relief with these dietary solutions for irritable bowel syndrome (IBS), it's important to get specific counsel from a healthcare provider or certified dietitian. By taking into account details like dietary demands, lifestyle choices, and particular symptoms, they may assist in developing a personalized strategy to meet those needs.

Foods to Eat on the IBS Diet

People who suffer from irritable bowel syndrome (IBS) may get relief from their symptoms by consuming the following foods.

Diets High in Soluble Fiber:

Soluble fiber can help those who suffer from irritable bowel syndrome. Soluble fiber, found in foods like oats, barley, bananas, apples, berries, and potatoes, can aid in bowel movement regulation and alleviate constipation.

Foods Rich in Probiotics:

The use of probiotics, also known as "good" bacteria, can be very helpful in maintaining digestive health. Yogurt, kefir, sauerkraut, and kimchi are excellent sources of probiotics, which may aid in restoring a healthy gut flora and alleviating gas and bloating.

Low-FODMAP Diet:

Irritable bowel syndrome (IBS) symptoms can be brought on by certain carbs called fermentable oligosaccharides, disaccharides, monosaccharides, and polyols. If you're experiencing symptoms like bloating and stomach pain, try eating low-FODMAP foods like rice, quinoa, zucchini, and lactose-free dairy products.

Lean Protein

Opt for lean protein sources like fish, tofu, and chicken instead of fatty or processed meats for a smoother digestive experience. Essential nutrients are provided by these proteins, and they won't make your IBS worse.

Ginger and Peppermint:

The natural digestive qualities of ginger and peppermint might alleviate stomach distress. Nausea and stomach cramps could be eased by ginger-infused foods or peppermint tea.

Eat Small Meals Often:

To avoid putting too much strain on the digestive system, it's best to eat smaller meals more often rather than three big ones. If this method works, it could make digestion easier and less likely to bring on IBS symptoms.

Common Food Triggers to Avoid on the IBS Diet

Recognizing and avoiding particular dietary triggers is essential for persons attempting to manage particular health concerns or preserve general wellness. Improving health outcomes can be greatly aided by learning about individual sensitivities and possible responses to specific chemicals. Some typical dietary triggers that people might want to steer clear of are:

Celiac disease and gluten sensitivity are both caused by the protein gluten, which is present in cereal grains such as wheat, barley, and rye. Some people experience gastrointestinal distress, inflammation, and other negative consequences after eating gluten-containing meals. As a result, rice flour or quinoa are common gluten-free options for people with celiac disease and other associated diseases.

For those who are lactose intolerant, the sugar in dairy products like milk, cheese, and yogurt might be difficult to digest. Symptoms like bloating, gas, and stomach pain can be avoided by avoiding certain dairy sources or opting for lactose-free alternatives.

Some people may be more sensitive to or allergic to processed foods because of the high concentrations of artificial additives, preservatives, and flavor enhancers in these meals. Reduce your risk of unpleasant reactions to synthetic additives by reading food labels and choosing full, unprocessed alternatives.

It is well-known that some people are very allergic to shellfish and some nuts. Those who suffer from severe food allergies should take extra precautions to avoid common allergens including peanuts, tree nuts, shrimp, and shellfish.

Obesity, diabetes, and inflammatory disorders are just a few of the health problems that may be exacerbated by refined sugars and the excessive intake of sugary foods and drinks. It may be helpful to limit sugar consumption by eating more whole fruits and using natural sweeteners like honey or maple syrup instead of sugary treats.

Foods that are very acidic, such tomatoes and citrus fruits, might cause acid reflux or make GERD symptoms worse in certain people. If you suffer from acid reflux, you can find relief by choosing low-acid options and avoiding acidic foods in the hours leading up to bedtime.

Caffeine, which is included in some sodas, coffees, and teas, can aggravate symptoms of anxiety, sleeplessness, and gastrointestinal problems in some people. One possible way to lessen the impact of these negative effects is to drink less coffee or use decaffeinated beverages.

Chapter 4: IBS RELIEF DIET RECIPES

IBS RELIEF BREAKFAST RECIPES

Banana Oat Pancakes

Ingredients:

1 ripe banana (ensure it's not overripe, as that can increase FODMAPs)

1 cup rolled oats

1/2 cup lactose-free milk or almond milk

1 teaspoon baking powder

1 tablespoon maple syrup (optional)

1 teaspoon vanilla extract

Pinch of salt

Cooking oil or butter for the pan

Instructions:

In a blender or food processor, combine the ripe banana, rolled oats, lactose-free milk, baking powder, maple syrup (if using), vanilla extract, and a pinch of salt. Blend until you achieve a smooth batter-like consistency.

Heat a non-stick skillet or griddle over medium heat and lightly grease it with cooking oil or butter.

Pour small amounts of the pancake batter onto the skillet to form pancakes of your desired size.

Cook the pancakes for 2-3 minutes on one side until bubbles form on the surface, then flip and cook for another 1-2 minutes on the other side until golden brown.

Remove the pancakes from the skillet and continue cooking the remaining batter in batches.

Serve the pancakes warm with toppings like fresh berries (low FODMAP fruits), a drizzle of maple syrup, or a dollop of lactose-free yogurt if tolerated.

Scrambled Tofu with Spinach and Tomatoes

Ingredients:

1 block firm tofu, drained and crumbled

1 cup fresh spinach, chopped

1 small tomato, diced

1 tablespoon olive oil

1 teaspoon turmeric

1/2 teaspoon paprika

Salt and pepper to taste

Chopped fresh herbs (parsley, chives) for garnish (optional)

Instructions:

Heat olive oil in a skillet over medium heat.

Add the crumbled tofu to the skillet and sprinkle turmeric and paprika over it. Cook for 3-4 minutes, stirring occasionally.

Add the chopped spinach and diced tomato to the skillet. Cook for an additional 2-3 minutes until the spinach wilts and the tomato softens.

Season with salt and pepper according to your taste.

Remove from heat and garnish with chopped fresh herbs if desired.

Serve the scrambled tofu warm on its own or with gluten-free toast or a side of low FODMAP fruits.

Croissant French Toast

Ingredients

4 large croissants, halved horizontally, left out overnight

3 large eggs

½ cup half-and-half

1 tablespoon white sugar

2 teaspoons vanilla extract

½ teaspoon ground cinnamon

¼ teaspoon salt

1 pinch ground nutmeg

2 tablespoons unsalted butter

INSTRUCTIONS

Preheat the oven to 200 degrees F (95 degrees C).

Whisk eggs, half-and-half, sugar, vanilla, cinnamon, salt, and nutmeg together in a shallow bowl. Dip each croissant half into egg mixture, one at a time, flipping it and lightly pressing down, until well coated.

Melt butter in a large skillet over medium heat; add four croissant halves, cut-side down. Fry until browned on both sides, turning once, 2 to 3 minutes per side. Transfer to the oven to keep warm while you cook the remaining croissants.

Serve warm with your favorite toppings.

Quinoa Breakfast Bowl

Ingredients:

1 cup cooked quinoa

1/2 cup lactose-free yogurt or coconut yogurt

1 tablespoon chia seeds

1/4 cup low FODMAP berries (such as blueberries, strawberries, or raspberries)

1 tablespoon sliced almonds or walnuts (optional)

1 tablespoon pure maple syrup (optional)

Cinnamon (optional)

Instructions:

In a bowl, place the cooked quinoa as the base.

Top the quinoa with lactose-free yogurt or coconut yogurt.

Sprinkle chia seeds over the yogurt layer.

Add low FODMAP berries and sliced almonds or walnuts on top.

Drizzle with a little pure maple syrup if desired for added sweetness or sprinkle some cinnamon for extra flavor.

Mix everything together before eating.

Peanut Butter Banana Rice Cakes

Ingredients:

2 rice cakes (choose low FODMAP rice cakes if available)

2 tablespoons natural peanut butter (look for varieties without added sugars or high FODMAP ingredients)

1 ripe banana, thinly sliced

Cinnamon (optional)

Chia seeds or pumpkin seeds (optional)

Instructions:

Spread a tablespoon of peanut butter evenly onto each rice cake.

Arrange the thinly sliced banana on top of the peanut butter layer.

Sprinkle a dash of cinnamon for added flavor if desired, and add a sprinkle of chia seeds or pumpkin seeds for extra texture and nutrients.

Serve immediately.

Veggie Omelette with Spinach and Peppers

Ingredients:

2-3 large eggs

1/4 cup chopped bell peppers (red, yellow, or green)

1/4 cup fresh spinach, chopped

1 tablespoon lactose-free cheese (optional)

1 tablespoon olive oil or butter

Salt and pepper to taste

Instructions:

In a bowl, whisk the eggs until well combined. Season with salt and pepper.

Heat olive oil or butter in a non-stick skillet over medium heat.

Add the chopped bell peppers to the skillet and sauté for 2-3 minutes until they start to soften.

Add the chopped spinach to the skillet and cook for an additional 1-2 minutes until wilted.

Pour the whisked eggs into the skillet, ensuring they cover the vegetables evenly.

Allow the omelette to cook for a few minutes until the edges start to set.

If using cheese, sprinkle it over one half of the omelette.

Gently fold the omelette in half using a spatula and cook for another minute or until the eggs are fully set and the cheese melts.

Slide the omelette onto a plate and serve warm.

Banana Almond Butter Toast

Ingredients:

2 slices of low FODMAP bread (such as sourdough or gluten-free bread)

2 tablespoons almond butter (check for no added high FODMAP ingredients)

1 ripe banana, sliced

Optional: A sprinkle of cinnamon or a drizzle of maple syrup (if tolerated)

Instructions:

Toast the bread: Toast the slices of bread to your desired level of doneness.

Spread almond butter: Once toasted, spread a generous layer of almond butter on each slice of bread.

Add banana slices: Arrange the banana slices on top of the almond butter layer.

Optional: Sprinkle a bit of cinnamon or drizzle a small amount of maple syrup over the bananas for extra flavor (if tolerated within your FODMAP limits).

Serve: Enjoy your delicious Banana Almond Butter Toast alongside a cup of herbal tea or your favorite low FODMAP beverage!

Chia Seed Pudding with Berries

Ingredients:

2 tablespoons chia seeds

1 cup lactose-free or almond milk

1/2 teaspoon vanilla extract

1 tablespoon maple syrup (optional, if tolerated)

1/2 cup mixed low FODMAP berries (such as strawberries, blueberries, raspberries)

Sliced almonds (for topping, if tolerated)

Instructions:

Mix chia seeds and milk: In a bowl or a jar, combine chia seeds, lactose-free or almond milk, vanilla extract, and maple syrup (if using). Stir well to ensure the chia seeds are evenly distributed. Let it sit for a couple of minutes.

Stir again: After a few minutes, stir the mixture again to prevent clumping of chia seeds. Then, cover and refrigerate it overnight or for at least 2-3 hours until it thickens into a pudding-like consistency.

Prepare the toppings: Wash and slice the mixed berries. If tolerated, you can also lightly toast some sliced almonds for added crunch.

Assemble: Once the chia pudding has thickened, spoon it into a bowl. Top it with the mixed berries and sliced almonds.

Enjoy: Your delicious and nutritious Low FODMAP Chia Seed Pudding with Berries is ready to be enjoyed as a satisfying breakfast!

Overnight Chia Seed Pudding

Ingredients:

1/4 cup chia seeds

1 cup lactose-free milk or almond milk

1/2 teaspoon vanilla extract

Low FODMAP sweetener such as maple syrup
or stevia (to taste)

Low FODMAP fruits (e.g., strawberries,
blueberries) for topping

Instructions:

In a bowl or jar, mix together the chia seeds,
lactose-free milk, vanilla extract, and sweetener
of choice. Stir well to combine.

Cover the bowl or jar and refrigerate it
overnight or for at least 4 hours to allow the chia

seeds to absorb the liquid and thicken into a pudding-like consistency.

Once the chia seed pudding has set, give it a good stir. If it's too thick, you can add a little more milk to reach your desired consistency.

Serve the chia seed pudding in a bowl or glass, and top it with low FODMAP fruits like strawberries or blueberries.

Overnight Oats with Peanut Butter and Banana

Ingredients:

1/2 cup rolled oats (certified gluten-free if needed)

1 cup lactose-free or almond milk

1 tablespoon chia seeds

1 tablespoon natural peanut butter (check for no added high FODMAP ingredients)

1 ripe banana, sliced

Optional: A sprinkle of cinnamon

Instructions:

Combine ingredients: In a jar or bowl, mix together the rolled oats, lactose-free or almond milk, chia seeds, and peanut butter. Stir well to ensure all ingredients are combined.

Add banana slices: Gently fold in the sliced banana into the oat mixture.

Cover and refrigerate: Cover the jar or bowl and refrigerate it overnight or for at least 4 hours to allow the oats and chia seeds to absorb the liquid and soften.

Optional: Before serving, sprinkle a bit of cinnamon for added flavor if desired.

Enjoy: Your delicious and creamy Low FODMAP Overnight Oats with Peanut Butter and Banana are ready to be enjoyed straight from the fridge in the morning!

Blueberry Banana Pancakes

Ingredients:

1 ripe banana, mashed

1 cup gluten-free flour (such as rice flour or oat flour)

1 teaspoon baking powder (check for no added high FODMAP ingredients)

1/2 cup lactose-free or almond milk

1/2 cup blueberries

1 tablespoon maple syrup (optional, if tolerated)

Cooking oil or cooking spray for the pan

Instructions:

Prepare the batter: In a mixing bowl, mash the ripe banana. Add the gluten-free flour, baking powder, lactose-free or almond milk, and maple syrup (if using). Mix until a smooth batter forms.

Fold in blueberries: Gently fold in the blueberries into the pancake batter.

Heat the pan: Heat a non-stick skillet or griddle over medium heat. Lightly grease the surface with cooking oil or cooking spray.

Cook the pancakes: Pour small portions of the batter onto the heated skillet to form pancakes. Cook until bubbles form on the surface, then flip and cook until golden brown on both sides.

Serve: Stack the pancakes on a plate and top with extra blueberries or a drizzle of maple syrup if desired.

Tofu Breakfast Burrito

Ingredients:

1 block firm tofu, drained and crumbled

1 tablespoon olive oil

1 teaspoon turmeric

1/2 teaspoon smoked paprika

Salt and pepper to taste

1 cup spinach

1/2 cup diced tomatoes (canned or fresh)

2-3 gluten-free tortillas (check for low FODMAP ingredients)

Optional toppings:

Sliced avocado

Low FODMAP salsa

Chopped fresh cilantro

Lactose-free cheese (if tolerated)

Instructions:

Prepare the tofu scramble: Heat olive oil in a skillet over medium heat. Add crumbled tofu, turmeric, smoked paprika, salt, and pepper. Cook for 5-7 minutes until the tofu starts to brown slightly.

Add vegetables: Add diced tomatoes and spinach to the skillet with the tofu. Cook for an additional 2-3 minutes until the spinach wilts and the tomatoes soften.

Warm the tortillas: Heat the gluten-free tortillas in a separate skillet or microwave for a few seconds to make them pliable.

Assemble the burritos: Spoon the tofu and vegetable mixture onto the center of each warmed tortilla. Add optional toppings like sliced avocado, low FODMAP salsa, chopped fresh cilantro, or lactose-free cheese if desired.

Roll the burritos: Fold the sides of the tortilla over the filling, then roll it up tightly to create a burrito.

Serve: Slice the burritos in half and serve them warm. They're a protein-packed and satisfying breakfast option that's easy to customize with your favorite low FODMAP toppings!

Turkey and Spinach Breakfast Wrap

Ingredients:

2 large eggs

2 slices low FODMAP deli turkey or cooked turkey breast

1/2 cup fresh spinach leaves

1 gluten-free or low FODMAP tortilla

Salt and pepper to taste

Olive oil or cooking spray

Instructions:

Heat a non-stick skillet over medium heat and lightly grease it with olive oil or cooking spray.

Crack the eggs into the skillet and scramble them until cooked through. Season with salt and pepper to taste.

Warm the tortilla in a separate skillet or microwave for a few seconds to make it pliable.

Lay the warmed tortilla flat and place the turkey slices on it, followed by the fresh spinach leaves.

Spoon the scrambled eggs onto the spinach.

Fold the sides of the tortilla over the filling and roll it up to create a wrap.

Optionally, you can warm the assembled wrap in the skillet for a minute or so to slightly crisp the tortilla and meld the flavors together.

Quinoa Breakfast Porridge

Ingredients:

1/2 cup quinoa, rinsed

1 cup lactose-free milk or almond milk

1/2 teaspoon ground cinnamon

1/4 teaspoon ground nutmeg

Low FODMAP sweetener such as maple syrup or stevia (to taste)

Low FODMAP fruits like sliced strawberries or blueberries for topping

Instructions:

In a saucepan, combine the rinsed quinoa and lactose-free milk.

Bring the mixture to a boil over medium-high heat, then reduce the heat to low and simmer, covered, for about 15-20 minutes or until the quinoa is cooked and the mixture has thickened, stirring occasionally.

Stir in the ground cinnamon and nutmeg.

Sweeten the porridge with your choice of low FODMAP sweetener to taste.

Once the porridge reaches your desired consistency, remove it from heat and let it sit for a minute or two to thicken further.

Serve the quinoa breakfast porridge in bowls and top it with low FODMAP fruits like sliced strawberries or blueberries.

Berry Smoothie Bowl

Ingredients:

1 cup mixed berries (blueberries, strawberries, raspberries)

1 ripe banana

1/2 cup lactose-free or almond milk

1 tablespoon chia seeds

Toppings: Sliced strawberries, blueberries, shredded coconut, sliced almonds (use FODMAP-friendly portions)

Instructions:

Prepare the base: In a blender, combine the mixed berries, banana, lactose-free or almond milk, and chia seeds. Blend until smooth and creamy.

Assemble the bowl: Pour the smoothie into a bowl.

Add toppings: Top the smoothie bowl with sliced strawberries, blueberries, shredded coconut, and sliced almonds (use FODMAP-friendly portions according to tolerance).

Grilled Chicken Salad with Lemon-Dijon Dressing

Ingredients:

For the Salad:

2 boneless, skinless chicken breasts

Mixed salad greens (lettuce, spinach, arugula, etc.)

1 cucumber, sliced

1 cup cherry tomatoes, halved

1/4 cup sliced red bell peppers

1/4 cup sliced carrots

1/4 cup sliced radishes (optional)

Olive oil for grilling

For the Lemon-Dijon Dressing:

2 tablespoons extra-virgin olive oil

1 tablespoon freshly squeezed lemon juice

1 teaspoon Dijon mustard

1 teaspoon honey or low FODMAP sweetener (optional)

Salt and pepper to taste

Instructions:

Preheat a grill or grill pan over medium-high heat.

Season the chicken breasts with salt and pepper and brush them lightly with olive oil.

Grill the chicken breasts for 5-7 minutes per side or until cooked through. Remove from the grill and let them rest for a few minutes before slicing.

In a small bowl, whisk together the extra-virgin olive oil, lemon juice, Dijon mustard, honey or sweetener (if using), salt, and pepper to make the dressing.

In a large salad bowl, combine the mixed greens, sliced cucumber, cherry tomatoes, red bell peppers, carrots, and radishes (if using).

Slice the grilled chicken breasts and add them to the salad.

Drizzle the lemon-Dijon dressing over the salad and toss gently to coat everything evenly.

Serve the grilled chicken salad immediately.

Lentil and Vegetable Soup

Ingredients:

1 cup dried green or brown lentils, rinsed

6 cups low FODMAP vegetable broth

1 cup diced carrots

1 cup diced zucchini

1 cup diced bell peppers (red, yellow, or green)

1 cup diced tomatoes (canned or fresh)

1 tablespoon garlic-infused oil (for low FODMAP option)

1 teaspoon dried thyme

Salt and pepper to taste

Fresh chopped parsley for garnish (optional)

Instructions:

Cook lentils: In a large pot, combine the rinsed lentils and low FODMAP vegetable broth. Bring to a boil, then reduce heat to a simmer. Cook for about 15-20 minutes or until the lentils are tender but not mushy.

Prepare vegetables: In a separate skillet, heat the garlic-infused oil over medium heat. Add the diced carrots, zucchini, bell peppers, and cook for 5-7 minutes until they start to soften.

Combine vegetables and lentils: Add the sautéed vegetables to the pot of cooked lentils.

Stir in the diced tomatoes and dried thyme. Simmer for an additional 10-15 minutes to let the flavors meld together.

Season and serve: Season the soup with salt and pepper to taste. Ladle the Low FODMAP Lentil and Vegetable Soup into bowls. Optionally, garnish with fresh chopped parsley for added flavor.

Tofu Buddha Bowl

Ingredients:

1 block firm tofu, drained and cubed

2 tablespoons garlic-infused oil (for low FODMAP option)

2 cups mixed greens (lettuce, spinach, arugula, etc.)

1 cup cooked quinoa or rice

1/2 cup shredded carrots

1/2 cup sliced cucumber

1/2 cup diced bell peppers (red, yellow, or green)

1/4 cup sliced radishes

1/4 cup chopped green tops of green onions (for those who tolerate them)

2 tablespoons sesame seeds (optional)

Low FODMAP dressing (such as a mix of olive oil, rice vinegar, and a touch of maple syrup)

Instructions:

Prepare the tofu: Heat 1 tablespoon of garlic-infused oil in a skillet over medium heat. Add the cubed tofu and cook until golden brown on all sides. Remove from heat and set aside.

Assemble the bowl: Divide the mixed greens, cooked quinoa or rice, shredded carrots, sliced cucumber, diced bell peppers, and sliced radishes into serving bowls.

Add tofu and toppings: Top the bowls with the cooked tofu cubes. If using, sprinkle the chopped green tops of green onions and sesame seeds over the bowls.

Drizzle dressing: Drizzle the Low FODMAP dressing over the Buddha bowls just before serving.

Mediterranean Quinoa Salad Wrap

Ingredients:

1 cup cooked quinoa

1/2 cup diced tomatoes (canned or fresh)

1/4 cup chopped cucumber

1/4 cup chopped red bell pepper

2 tablespoons chopped Kalamata olives (check for no added high FODMAP ingredients)

2 tablespoons chopped fresh parsley

1 tablespoon olive oil

1 tablespoon fresh lemon juice

Salt and pepper to taste

Low FODMAP wrap or tortilla (check for low FODMAP ingredients)

Mixed greens or lettuce leaves

Instructions:

Prepare the quinoa salad: In a bowl, combine the cooked quinoa, diced tomatoes, chopped cucumber, chopped red bell pepper, chopped Kalamata olives, chopped fresh parsley, olive oil, and fresh lemon juice. Season with salt and pepper to taste. Mix well.

Assemble the wrap: Lay a low FODMAP wrap or tortilla on a clean surface. Place a few mixed greens or lettuce leaves on the wrap.

Add quinoa salad: Spoon the prepared Mediterranean quinoa salad onto the greens in the center of the wrap.

Fold and roll: Fold in the sides of the wrap, then roll it up tightly from the bottom to enclose the filling, creating a wrap.

Slice and serve: Carefully slice the wrap in half if desired, and serve immediately.

Sushi Bowl

Ingredients:

1 cup cooked sushi rice (or substitute with quinoa for a different twist)

1/2 cup sliced cucumber

1/2 cup sliced red bell pepper

1/2 cup sliced carrots

1/2 cup sliced radishes

1/2 cup diced firm tofu

1 tablespoon sesame seeds (optional)

2 tablespoons low-sodium soy sauce (for gluten-free, ensure it's low FODMAP)

1 tablespoon rice vinegar

1 tablespoon maple syrup

1 teaspoon sesame oil

Nori strips (seaweed sheets), sliced into thin strips for garnish (optional)

Instructions:

Prepare the dressing: In a small bowl, whisk together the low-sodium soy sauce, rice vinegar, maple syrup, and sesame oil. Set aside.

Assemble the bowl: Divide the cooked sushi rice or quinoa into serving bowls. Arrange the sliced cucumber, red bell pepper, carrots, radishes, and diced tofu on top of the rice in separate sections.

Drizzle the dressing: Drizzle the prepared dressing over the ingredients in the bowl. Sprinkle sesame seeds on top if using.

Garnish with nori strips: If desired, garnish the bowls with sliced nori strips for added flavor.

Mexican Quinoa Bowl

Ingredients:

1 cup cooked quinoa

1 cup diced tomatoes (canned or fresh)

1 cup cooked and drained black beans (canned, rinsed)

1/2 cup sliced bell peppers (red, yellow, or green)

1/2 cup sliced cucumber

1/4 cup chopped fresh cilantro

2 tablespoons sliced black olives (check for no added high FODMAP ingredients)

1 tablespoon olive oil

1 tablespoon fresh lime juice

1 teaspoon ground cumin

Salt and pepper to taste

Optional: Sliced jalapeños (if tolerated)

Instructions:

Prepare the quinoa: Cook quinoa according to package instructions and set aside.

Prepare the vegetables and beans: In a bowl, combine the diced tomatoes, cooked black beans, sliced bell peppers, sliced cucumber, chopped fresh cilantro, and sliced black olives.

Make the dressing: In a small bowl, whisk together the olive oil, fresh lime juice, ground cumin, salt, and pepper.

Assemble the bowl: Divide the cooked quinoa into serving bowls. Top with the prepared vegetable and bean mixture.

Drizzle with dressing: Drizzle the dressing over the ingredients in the bowl.

Optional: If desired, add sliced jalapeños for a bit of heat.

Veggie Stir-Fry Noodle Bowl

Ingredients:

8 oz (about 225g) rice noodles (check for low FODMAP ingredients)

2 tablespoons garlic-infused oil (for low FODMAP option)

1 block firm tofu, drained and cubed

2 cups mixed low FODMAP vegetables (bell peppers, carrots, bok choy, etc.), sliced

1 tablespoon low-sodium soy sauce (for gluten-free, ensure it's low FODMAP)

1 tablespoon rice vinegar

1 tablespoon maple syrup

Sesame seeds for garnish (optional)

Chopped green tops of green onions (for those
who tolerate them) for garnish (optional)

Instructions:

Prepare the rice noodles: Cook the rice noodles
according to package instructions. Drain and
set aside.

Cook the tofu: Heat 1 tablespoon of garlic-
infused oil in a large skillet or wok over medium
heat. Add the cubed tofu and cook until golden

brown on all sides. Remove the tofu from the skillet and set it aside.

Stir-fry the vegetables: In the same skillet, add the remaining tablespoon of garlic-infused oil if needed. Add the mixed vegetables and stir-fry for 3-4 minutes until they are tender-crisp.

Combine tofu and vegetables: Return the cooked tofu to the skillet with the vegetables.

Make the sauce: In a small bowl, whisk together the low-sodium soy sauce, rice vinegar, and maple syrup. Pour the sauce over the tofu and vegetables in the skillet. Toss everything together until well coated and heated through.

Assemble the noodle bowls: Divide the cooked rice noodles into serving bowls. Top with the tofu and vegetable stir-fry.

Garnish and serve: Garnish with sesame seeds and chopped green tops of green onions if using.

Quinoa and Roasted Vegetable Salad

Ingredients:

1 cup quinoa, rinsed

2 cups low FODMAP vegetable broth or water

2 cups mixed low FODMAP vegetables (bell peppers, zucchini, carrots, eggplant), diced

2 tablespoons olive oil

Salt and pepper to taste

1 tablespoon fresh lemon juice

2 tablespoons chopped fresh parsley

Optional: Feta cheese (if tolerated)

Instructions:

Prepare the quinoa: In a saucepan, combine the rinsed quinoa and low FODMAP vegetable broth or water. Bring to a boil, then reduce heat to low, cover, and simmer for 15-20 minutes or until the quinoa is cooked and the liquid is absorbed. Set aside.

Roast the vegetables: Preheat the oven to 400°F (200°C). Toss the diced mixed vegetables with olive oil, salt, and pepper. Spread them on a baking sheet and roast for about 20-25 minutes or until they're tender and slightly caramelized.

Remove from the oven and let them cool slightly.

Assemble the salad: In a large mixing bowl, combine the cooked quinoa and roasted vegetables. Add fresh lemon juice and chopped parsley. Toss gently until well mixed.

Optional: If desired and tolerated, crumble feta cheese on top of the salad for added flavor.

Serve: This Low FODMAP Quinoa and Roasted Vegetable Salad can be served warm or at room temperature. It's a hearty and flavorful lunch option that's packed with nutrients and customizable with your favorite low FODMAP veggies!

Thai Peanut Tofu Bowl

Ingredients:

1 block firm tofu, drained and cubed

2 tablespoons garlic-infused oil (for low FODMAP option)

1 cup cooked rice or quinoa

2 cups mixed low FODMAP vegetables (bell peppers, carrots, zucchini), sliced

1/4 cup chopped peanuts (check for no added high FODMAP ingredients)

Fresh cilantro for garnish

Lime wedges for serving

For the peanut sauce:

2 tablespoons peanut butter (ensure no high FODMAP ingredients)

2 tablespoons low-sodium soy sauce (for gluten-free, ensure it's low FODMAP)

1 tablespoon maple syrup

1 tablespoon rice vinegar

1 teaspoon sesame oil

Water (to adjust consistency)

Instructions:

Prepare the peanut sauce: In a small bowl, whisk together the peanut butter, low-sodium soy sauce, maple syrup, rice vinegar, and sesame oil. Add water gradually to reach the desired consistency. Set aside.

Cook the tofu: Heat 1 tablespoon of garlic-infused oil in a skillet over medium heat. Add the cubed tofu and cook until golden brown on all sides. Remove the tofu from the skillet and set it aside.

Stir-fry the vegetables: In the same skillet, add the remaining tablespoon of garlic-infused oil if needed. Stir-fry the mixed vegetables for 3-4 minutes until they are tender-crisp.

Assemble the bowl: Divide the cooked rice or quinoa into serving bowls. Top with the stir-fried vegetables and cooked tofu.

Drizzle with peanut sauce: Drizzle the prepared peanut sauce over the ingredients in the bowl.

Garnish and serve: Garnish with chopped peanuts, fresh cilantro, and serve with lime wedges on the side.

Quinoa and Vegetable Stir-Fry

Ingredients:

1 cup quinoa, rinsed

2 cups water or low-sodium vegetable broth

1 tablespoon olive oil

1 bell pepper, sliced

1 zucchini, sliced

1 cup sliced carrots

1 cup broccoli florets

2 cloves garlic, minced

2 tablespoons low-sodium soy sauce or tamari (gluten-free option)

1 tablespoon rice vinegar

1 teaspoon sesame oil (optional)

Salt and pepper to taste

Chopped green onions (green parts only, for garnish)

Instructions:

In a saucepan, combine the rinsed quinoa and water or vegetable broth. Bring it to a boil, then reduce heat to low, cover, and simmer for about 15-20 minutes or until the liquid is absorbed and the quinoa is cooked. Set aside.

Heat olive oil in a large skillet or wok over medium-high heat.

Add the sliced bell pepper, zucchini, carrots, and broccoli to the skillet. Stir-fry for 4-5 minutes until the vegetables start to soften but are still crisp.

Add the minced garlic and continue stir-frying for another minute.

In a small bowl, mix together the low-sodium soy sauce or tamari, rice vinegar, and sesame oil (if using).

Pour the sauce over the vegetables in the skillet and stir to coat evenly. Cook for an additional 1-2 minutes.

Season with salt and pepper to taste.

Serve the vegetable stir-fry over a bed of cooked quinoa and garnish with chopped green onions.

Baked Salmon with Roasted Vegetables

Ingredients:

2 salmon fillets

2 tablespoons olive oil

1 teaspoon paprika

1 teaspoon dried thyme

Salt and pepper to taste

1 zucchini, sliced

1 red bell pepper, sliced

1 yellow bell pepper, sliced

1 small eggplant, diced

1 tablespoon balsamic vinegar

Fresh parsley for garnish (optional)

Instructions:

Preheat your oven to 400°F (200°C).

Place the salmon fillets on a baking sheet lined with parchment paper.

In a small bowl, mix together 1 tablespoon of olive oil, paprika, dried thyme, salt, and pepper. Brush this mixture over the salmon fillets.

In a separate bowl, toss the sliced zucchini, red and yellow bell peppers, and diced eggplant with the remaining tablespoon of olive oil and balsamic vinegar until coated.

Spread the vegetables on a separate baking sheet.

Place both baking sheets in the oven. Bake the salmon for 12-15 minutes or until it flakes easily with a fork, and roast the vegetables for 20-25 minutes or until they are tender and slightly caramelized.

Once done, remove the salmon and vegetables from the oven.

Serve the baked salmon alongside the roasted vegetables, garnished with fresh parsley if desired.

Veggie and Tofu Rice Paper Rolls

Ingredients:

Rice paper wrappers (check for low FODMAP ingredients)

1 block firm tofu, drained and cut into thin strips

1 cup mixed low FODMAP vegetables (lettuce, carrots, bell peppers, cucumber), julienned

Fresh herbs like cilantro or mint leaves

Low FODMAP dipping sauce (such as a combination of tamari, sesame oil, and a touch of maple syrup)

Instructions:

Prepare the tofu: Heat a non-stick skillet over medium heat. Add a little oil and cook the tofu strips until they're golden brown on both sides. Remove from heat and set aside.

Prepare the vegetables and herbs: Julienne the mixed vegetables and set them aside. Wash and prepare the fresh herbs.

Soften rice paper wrappers: Fill a large shallow dish or bowl with warm water. Dip one rice paper wrapper into the warm water for about 15-20 seconds until it softens. Place it on a clean, damp kitchen towel or a plate.

Assemble the rolls: Place a few strips of tofu, a handful of julienned vegetables, and some fresh herbs (cilantro or mint leaves) in the center of the softened rice paper wrapper, leaving some space on the sides. Fold the sides of the wrapper over the filling, then tightly roll it up from the bottom to enclose the filling.

Repeat and serve: Continue assembling the rolls with the remaining ingredients. Serve the Low FODMAP Veggie and Tofu Rice Paper Rolls with the low FODMAP dipping sauce.

Quinoa Stuffed Bell Peppers

Ingredients:

4 bell peppers (red, yellow, or green)

1 cup quinoa, rinsed

2 cups low FODMAP vegetable broth or water

1 tablespoon olive oil

1 cup mixed low FODMAP vegetables (such as zucchini, carrots, spinach), diced

1/2 cup diced tomatoes (canned or fresh)

1 teaspoon dried oregano

Salt and pepper to taste

Optional: Grated lactose-free cheese (if tolerated)

Instructions:

Prepare the bell peppers: Preheat the oven to 375°F (190°C). Cut the tops off the bell peppers and remove the seeds and membranes from the insides. Place the bell peppers in a baking dish, cut-side up.

Cook quinoa: In a saucepan, combine the rinsed quinoa and low FODMAP vegetable broth or water. Bring to a boil, then reduce heat to low, cover, and simmer for 15-20 minutes or until the quinoa is cooked and the liquid is absorbed.

Prepare the filling: In a skillet, heat olive oil over medium heat. Add the diced mixed vegetables and sauté for a few minutes until they start to soften. Add the diced tomatoes, dried oregano, salt, and pepper. Cook for an additional 2-3 minutes.

Combine quinoa and filling: In a mixing bowl, combine the cooked quinoa with the sautéed vegetable mixture. Mix well to combine all the flavors.

Stuff the bell peppers: Spoon the quinoa and vegetable mixture into the hollowed-out bell peppers, packing it gently. If desired, top each stuffed bell pepper with a sprinkle of grated lactose-free cheese.

Bake: Cover the baking dish with foil and bake in the preheated oven for 25-30 minutes, or until the bell peppers are tender.

Serve: Remove from the oven and let them cool slightly before serving. Enjoy these flavorful and satisfying Low FODMAP Quinoa Stuffed Bell Peppers!

Tofu and Veggie Stir-Fry with Brown Rice

Ingredients:

1 block firm tofu, drained and cubed

2 tablespoons garlic-infused oil (for low FODMAP option)

2 cups mixed low FODMAP vegetables (bell peppers, bok choy, carrots, snow peas, etc.), sliced

1-inch piece of fresh ginger, grated

2 tablespoons low-sodium soy sauce (for gluten-free, ensure it's low FODMAP)

Salt and pepper to taste

2 cups cooked brown rice

Instructions:

Prepare the tofu: Heat 1 tablespoon of garlic-infused oil in a large skillet or wok over medium heat. Add the cubed tofu and cook until golden brown on all sides, stirring occasionally. Remove the tofu from the skillet and set it aside.

Stir-fry the vegetables: In the same skillet, add the remaining garlic-infused oil if needed. Add the mixed vegetables and grated ginger. Stir-fry for 3-4 minutes until the vegetables are tender-crisp.

Add tofu and seasoning: Return the cooked tofu to the skillet with the vegetables. Pour in the low-sodium soy sauce. Season with salt and pepper to taste. Toss everything together until well combined.

Serve: Divide the cooked brown rice into serving bowls or plates. Top with the Tofu and Veggie Stir-Fry mixture.

Quinoa Salad with Lemon-Herb Dressing

Ingredients:

For the Salad:

1 cup quinoa, rinsed

2 cups low-sodium vegetable broth or water

1 cup diced cucumber

1 cup halved cherry tomatoes

1/2 cup chopped red bell pepper

1/4 cup chopped fresh parsley

1/4 cup chopped fresh mint leaves

1/4 cup crumbled feta cheese (optional)

Salt and pepper to taste

For the Lemon-Herb Dressing:

1/4 cup extra-virgin olive oil

Zest and juice of 1 lemon

1 tablespoon chopped fresh parsley

1 tablespoon chopped fresh mint leaves

1 clove garlic, minced (optional)

Salt and pepper to taste

Instructions:

In a saucepan, combine the rinsed quinoa and vegetable broth or water. Bring it to a boil, then reduce heat to low, cover, and simmer for 15-20 minutes or until the liquid is absorbed and the quinoa is cooked. Fluff with a fork and let it cool.

In a large mixing bowl, combine the cooked and cooled quinoa with diced cucumber, cherry tomatoes, chopped red bell pepper, chopped parsley, and chopped mint. Mix well.

If using, add crumbled feta cheese to the salad and gently toss.

In a small bowl, whisk together the extra-virgin olive oil, lemon zest, lemon juice, chopped parsley, chopped mint, minced garlic (if using), salt, and pepper to make the dressing.

Drizzle the lemon-herb dressing over the quinoa salad and toss gently to coat everything evenly.

Season with additional salt and pepper if needed.

Serve the quinoa salad at room temperature or chilled.

IBS RELIEF DINNER RECIPES

Lemon Herb Baked Cod

Ingredients:

4 cod fillets

2 tablespoons olive oil

2 tablespoons fresh lemon juice

Zest of 1 lemon

2 cloves garlic, minced

1 teaspoon dried thyme

1 teaspoon dried parsley

Salt and pepper to taste

Sliced lemon for garnish

Instructions:

Preheat your oven to 375°F (190°C).

In a small bowl, mix together the olive oil, fresh lemon juice, lemon zest, minced garlic, dried thyme, dried parsley, salt, and pepper.

Place the cod fillets in a baking dish.

Pour the prepared mixture over the cod, ensuring the fillets are evenly coated.

Place a few slices of lemon on top of each fillet for added flavor.

Cover the baking dish with foil and let the fish marinate in the refrigerator for at least 30 minutes.

Once marinated, bake the cod in the preheated oven for about 15-20 minutes or until the fish is cooked through and flakes easily with a fork.

Optionally, remove the foil for the last few minutes of baking to lightly brown the top.

Serve the lemon herb baked cod with your choice of side dishes such as steamed vegetables, quinoa, or a side salad.

Tofu and Vegetable Stir-Fry

Ingredients:

1 block firm tofu, drained and cubed

2 tablespoons garlic-infused oil (for low FODMAP option)

2 cups mixed low FODMAP vegetables (bell peppers, carrots, bok choy, etc.), sliced

1 tablespoon low-sodium soy sauce (for gluten-free, ensure it's low FODMAP)

1 tablespoon rice vinegar

1 tablespoon maple syrup

Sesame seeds for garnish (optional)

Cooked rice or quinoa for serving

Instructions:

Prepare the tofu: Heat 1 tablespoon of garlic-infused oil in a skillet over medium heat. Add the cubed tofu and cook until golden brown on all sides. Remove the tofu from the skillet and set it aside.

Stir-fry the vegetables: In the same skillet, add the remaining tablespoon of garlic-infused oil if needed. Stir-fry the mixed vegetables for 3-4 minutes until they are tender-crisp.

Combine tofu and vegetables: Return the cooked tofu to the skillet with the vegetables.

Make the sauce: In a small bowl, mix together the low-sodium soy sauce, rice vinegar, and maple syrup. Pour the sauce over the tofu and vegetables in the skillet. Toss everything together until well coated and heated through.

Serve: Serve the Stir-Fried Tofu and Vegetables over cooked rice or quinoa. Garnish with sesame seeds if desired.

Veggie and Tofu Stir-Fry

Ingredients:

1 block firm tofu, drained and cubed

2 tablespoons garlic-infused oil (for low FODMAP option)

2 cups mixed low FODMAP vegetables (bell peppers, carrots, zucchini), sliced

1 tablespoon low-sodium soy sauce (for gluten-free, ensure it's low FODMAP)

1 tablespoon rice vinegar

1 tablespoon maple syrup

Cooked rice or quinoa for serving

Instructions:

Prepare the tofu: Heat 1 tablespoon of garlic-infused oil in a skillet over medium heat. Add the cubed tofu and cook until golden brown on all sides. Remove the tofu from the skillet and set aside.

Stir-fry the vegetables: In the same skillet, add the remaining tablespoon of garlic-infused oil if needed. Stir-fry the mixed vegetables for 3-4 minutes until they are tender-crisp.

Combine tofu and vegetables: Return the cooked tofu to the skillet with the vegetables.

Make the sauce: In a small bowl, mix together the low-sodium soy sauce, rice vinegar, and maple syrup. Pour the sauce over the tofu and vegetables in the skillet. Toss everything together until well coated and heated through.

Serve: Serve the Veggie and Tofu Stir-Fry over cooked rice or quinoa.

Mexican Quinoa Bowl

Ingredients:

1 cup quinoa, rinsed

2 cups low FODMAP vegetable broth or water

1 cup diced tomatoes (canned or fresh)

1 cup cooked and drained black beans (canned, rinsed)

1/2 cup sliced bell peppers (red, yellow, or green)

1/2 cup sliced cucumber

1/4 cup chopped fresh cilantro

2 tablespoons sliced black olives (check for no added high FODMAP ingredients)

1 tablespoon olive oil

1 tablespoon fresh lime juice

1 teaspoon ground cumin

Salt and pepper to taste

Instructions:

Prepare the quinoa: Cook quinoa according to package instructions using low FODMAP vegetable broth or water. Set aside.

Prepare the vegetables: In a bowl, combine diced tomatoes, black beans, sliced bell peppers, sliced cucumber, chopped fresh cilantro, and sliced black olives.

Make the dressing: In a small bowl, whisk together olive oil, fresh lime juice, ground cumin, salt, and pepper.

Assemble the bowl: Divide the cooked quinoa into serving bowls. Top with the prepared vegetable and bean mixture.

Drizzle with dressing: Drizzle the dressing over the ingredients in the bowl.

Lentil and Spinach Curry

Ingredients:

1 cup dried lentils, rinsed

4 cups low FODMAP vegetable broth

1 tablespoon garlic-infused oil (for low FODMAP option)

1 cup diced tomatoes (canned or fresh)

2 cups fresh spinach

1 teaspoon ground cumin

1 teaspoon ground coriander

1 teaspoon turmeric

1/2 teaspoon paprika

Salt and pepper to taste

Cooked rice for serving

Instructions:

Cook the lentils: In a pot, combine the rinsed lentils and low FODMAP vegetable broth. Bring to a boil, then reduce heat to a simmer. Cook for 20-25 minutes or until the lentils are tender.

Prepare the curry: In a separate large skillet, heat garlic-infused oil over medium heat. Add diced tomatoes, ground cumin, ground coriander, turmeric, paprika, salt, and pepper. Cook for a few minutes until the tomatoes soften.

Combine ingredients: Add the cooked lentils (with any remaining broth) to the skillet with the tomato mixture. Stir well to combine. Add fresh spinach and continue to cook for another 3-4 minutes until the spinach wilts.

Serve: Serve the lentil and spinach curry over cooked rice.

Eggplant & Tofu Stir-Fry

Ingredients:

1 large eggplant, diced

1 block firm tofu, drained and cubed

2 tablespoons garlic-infused oil (for low FODMAP option)

2 cups mixed low FODMAP vegetables (bell peppers, carrots, bok choy), sliced

1 tablespoon low-sodium soy sauce (for gluten-free, ensure it's low FODMAP)

1 tablespoon rice vinegar

1 tablespoon maple syrup

Cooked rice or quinoa for serving

Instructions:

Prepare the eggplant: Place the diced eggplant in a colander and sprinkle it with salt. Let it sit for 20-30 minutes to draw out excess moisture. Rinse and pat dry.

Prepare the tofu: Heat 1 tablespoon of garlic-infused oil in a skillet over medium heat. Add the cubed tofu and cook until golden brown on all sides. Remove the tofu from the skillet and set it aside.

Stir-fry the vegetables: In the same skillet, add the remaining tablespoon of garlic-infused oil if needed. Add the mixed vegetables and diced eggplant. Stir-fry for 5-7 minutes until they are tender.

Combine tofu and vegetables: Return the cooked tofu to the skillet with the vegetables.

Make the sauce: In a small bowl, mix together the low-sodium soy sauce, rice vinegar, and maple syrup. Pour the sauce over the tofu and vegetables in the skillet. Toss everything together until well coated and heated through.

Serve: Serve the Eggplant & Tofu Stir-Fry over cooked rice or quinoa.

Low FODMAP Lentil and Vegetable Soup

Ingredients:

1 cup dried green lentils, rinsed

4 cups low FODMAP vegetable broth

1 cup diced carrots

1 cup diced zucchini

1 cup diced potatoes

1 cup chopped spinach

1 tablespoon garlic-infused oil (for low FODMAP option)

1 teaspoon dried thyme

1 teaspoon dried oregano

Salt and pepper to taste

Fresh parsley for garnish

Instructions:

Cook the lentils: In a pot, combine the rinsed lentils and low FODMAP vegetable broth. Bring to a boil, then reduce heat to a simmer. Cook for about 20-25 minutes or until the lentils are tender.

Prepare the vegetables: In a separate skillet, heat garlic-infused oil over medium heat. Add diced carrots, zucchini, potatoes, and cook for about 5 minutes until slightly softened.

Combine ingredients: Add the cooked vegetables to the pot with the lentils. Stir in dried thyme, dried oregano, salt, and pepper. Simmer for an additional 10-15 minutes.

Add spinach and season: Stir in chopped spinach and simmer for a few more minutes until the spinach wilts. Adjust seasoning if needed.

Serve: Ladle the Low FODMAP Lentil and Vegetable Soup into bowls, garnish with fresh parsley, and serve warm.

Quinoa and Veggie Stir-Fry

Ingredients:

1 cup quinoa, rinsed

2 cups low FODMAP vegetable broth or water

1 block firm tofu, drained and cubed

2 tablespoons garlic-infused oil (for low FODMAP option)

2 cups mixed low FODMAP vegetables (bell peppers, carrots, bok choy, etc.), sliced

1 tablespoon low-sodium soy sauce (for gluten-free, ensure it's low FODMAP)

1 tablespoon rice vinegar

1 tablespoon maple syrup

Sesame seeds for garnish (optional)

Instructions:

Prepare the quinoa: In a saucepan, combine the rinsed quinoa and low FODMAP vegetable broth or water. Bring to a boil, then reduce heat to low, cover, and simmer for 15-20 minutes or until the quinoa is cooked and the liquid is absorbed. Set aside.

Prepare the tofu: Heat 1 tablespoon of garlic-infused oil in a skillet over medium heat. Add the cubed tofu and cook until golden brown on all sides. Remove the tofu from the skillet and set it aside.

Stir-fry the vegetables: In the same skillet, add the remaining tablespoon of garlic-infused oil if needed. Stir-fry the mixed vegetables for 3-4 minutes until they are tender-crisp.

Combine tofu and vegetables: Return the cooked tofu to the skillet with the vegetables.

Make the sauce: In a small bowl, mix together the low-sodium soy sauce, rice vinegar, and maple syrup. Pour the sauce over the tofu and vegetables in the skillet. Toss everything together until well coated and heated through.

Serve: Serve the Stir-Fried Quinoa and Vegetables with tofu over cooked quinoa. Garnish with sesame seeds if desired.

Turkey and Vegetable Stir-Fry

Ingredients:

1 pound ground turkey

2 tablespoons olive oil

2 cups mixed vegetables (such as bell peppers, zucchini, carrots, broccoli)

2 tablespoons low-sodium soy sauce or tamari (gluten-free option)

1 tablespoon rice vinegar

1 teaspoon grated ginger

2 cloves garlic, minced

Salt and pepper to taste

Cooked rice or quinoa for serving

Instructions:

Heat one tablespoon of olive oil in a large skillet or wok over medium-high heat.

Add the ground turkey to the skillet and cook until browned, breaking it into crumbles as it cooks. Remove the cooked turkey from the skillet and set it aside.

In the same skillet, add the remaining tablespoon of olive oil and stir-fry the mixed vegetables until they start to soften but still have a slight crunch.

Add the grated ginger and minced garlic to the skillet and cook for an additional minute.

Return the cooked turkey to the skillet with the vegetables.

In a small bowl, mix together the low-sodium soy sauce or tamari, rice vinegar, and a pinch of salt and pepper.

Pour the sauce over the turkey and vegetables in the skillet. Stir-fry for a few more minutes until everything is heated through and coated with the sauce.

Serve the turkey and vegetable stir-fry over cooked rice or quinoa.

Baked Chicken with Roasted Vegetables

Ingredients:

4 boneless, skinless chicken breasts

2 tablespoons olive oil

2 cloves garlic, minced

1 teaspoon dried thyme

1 teaspoon dried rosemary

1 teaspoon paprika

Salt and pepper to taste

2 cups mixed vegetables (bell peppers, carrots, zucchini, etc.), chopped

Cooking spray

Instructions:

Preheat your oven to 400°F (200°C).

In a small bowl, mix together the olive oil, minced garlic, dried thyme, dried rosemary, paprika, salt, and pepper.

Place the chicken breasts in a baking dish. Brush each breast with the prepared olive oil and herb mixture, ensuring they're well coated.

In a separate bowl, toss the mixed vegetables with a little olive oil, salt, and pepper.

Arrange the seasoned vegetables around the chicken breasts in the baking dish.

Lightly coat the vegetables with cooking spray to prevent them from drying out while baking.

Bake in the preheated oven for 20-25 minutes or until the chicken is cooked through (internal temperature should reach 165°F or 74°C) and the vegetables are tender, stirring the vegetables halfway through.

Once done, remove from the oven and let it rest for a few minutes before serving.

Shrimp and Vegetable Stir-Fry

Ingredients:

1 pound shrimp, peeled and deveined

2 tablespoons olive oil

2 cups mixed vegetables (such as bell peppers, snap peas, carrots, broccoli)

2 cloves garlic, minced

1 tablespoon grated ginger

2 tablespoons low-sodium soy sauce or tamari (gluten-free option)

1 tablespoon rice vinegar

1 teaspoon sesame oil (optional)

Salt and pepper to taste

Cooked rice or quinoa for serving

Instructions:

Heat one tablespoon of olive oil in a large skillet or wok over medium-high heat.

Add the shrimp to the skillet and cook until they turn pink and are cooked through. Remove the cooked shrimp from the skillet and set them aside.

In the same skillet, add the remaining tablespoon of olive oil and stir-fry the mixed vegetables until they're tender-crisp.

Add the minced garlic and grated ginger to the skillet, stirring constantly for about a minute.

Return the cooked shrimp to the skillet with the vegetables.

In a small bowl, mix together the low-sodium soy sauce or tamari, rice vinegar, and sesame oil (if using). Pour the sauce over the shrimp and vegetables.

Stir-fry everything together for a few more minutes until heated through and coated with the sauce.

Season with salt and pepper to taste.

Serve the shrimp and vegetable stir-fry over cooked rice or quinoa.

Baked Turkey Meatballs with Zucchini Noodles

Ingredients:

For the Turkey Meatballs:

1 pound ground turkey

1/4 cup gluten-free breadcrumbs or almond flour

1 egg

2 tablespoons chopped fresh parsley

1 teaspoon dried oregano

1 teaspoon paprika

Salt and pepper to taste

For the Zucchini Noodles:

4 medium zucchinis, spiralized into noodles

2 tablespoons olive oil

2 cloves garlic, minced

Salt and pepper to taste

Freshly grated Parmesan cheese for garnish (optional)

Instructions:

Turkey Meatballs:

Preheat your oven to 400°F (200°C).

In a mixing bowl, combine the ground turkey, gluten-free breadcrumbs or almond flour, egg, chopped parsley, dried oregano, paprika, salt, and pepper. Mix until well combined.

Form the mixture into meatballs of your desired size and place them on a baking sheet lined with parchment paper.

Bake the meatballs in the preheated oven for 15-20 minutes or until they are cooked through and browned.

Zucchini Noodles:

While the meatballs are baking, heat olive oil in a large skillet over medium heat.

Add minced garlic to the skillet and cook for about 1 minute until fragrant.

Add the spiralized zucchini noodles to the skillet and toss them in the garlic oil. Cook for

2-3 minutes until the noodles are just tender but not overly soft.

Season the zucchini noodles with salt and pepper to taste.

Remove the zucchini noodles from heat.

Assembly:

Serve the baked turkey meatballs alongside the cooked zucchini noodles.

Optionally, garnish with freshly grated Parmesan cheese before serving.

Baked Salmon with Herb Quinoa

Ingredients:

For the Baked Salmon:

4 salmon fillets

2 tablespoons olive oil

2 tablespoons freshly squeezed lemon juice

2 cloves garlic, minced

1 teaspoon dried dill

1 teaspoon dried parsley

Salt and pepper to taste

Lemon wedges for serving

For the Herb Quinoa:

1 cup quinoa, rinsed

2 cups low-sodium vegetable broth or water

1 tablespoon olive oil

2 tablespoons chopped fresh parsley

1 tablespoon chopped fresh dill

Salt and pepper to taste

Instructions:

Baked Salmon:

Preheat your oven to 375°F (190°C).

Place the salmon fillets on a baking sheet lined with parchment paper.

In a small bowl, mix together the olive oil, lemon juice, minced garlic, dried dill, dried parsley, salt, and pepper.

Brush the salmon fillets with the prepared mixture, ensuring they are well coated.

Bake the salmon in the preheated oven for about 12-15 minutes or until the fish is cooked through and flakes easily with a fork.

Once done, remove the salmon from the oven and serve with lemon wedges.

Herb Quinoa:

In a saucepan, combine the rinsed quinoa and low-sodium vegetable broth or water. Bring it to a boil, then reduce heat to low, cover, and simmer for 15-20 minutes or until the liquid is absorbed and the quinoa is cooked.

Fluff the cooked quinoa with a fork.

In a bowl, combine the cooked quinoa with olive oil, chopped fresh parsley, chopped fresh dill, salt, and pepper. Mix well.

Serving:

Serve the baked salmon alongside a portion of herb quinoa.

Optionally, add a squeeze of lemon over the salmon before serving.

Lemon Herb Chicken with Roasted Potatoes

Ingredients:

For the Lemon Herb Chicken:

4 boneless, skinless chicken breasts

2 tablespoons olive oil

Zest and juice of 1 lemon

2 cloves garlic, minced

1 teaspoon dried thyme

1 teaspoon dried rosemary

Salt and pepper to taste

For the Roasted Potatoes:

4 medium-sized potatoes, washed and diced into cubes

2 tablespoons olive oil

1 teaspoon paprika

1 teaspoon dried parsley

Salt and pepper to taste

Instructions:

Lemon Herb Chicken:

Preheat your oven to 375°F (190°C).

In a bowl, combine the olive oil, lemon zest, lemon juice, minced garlic, dried thyme, dried rosemary, salt, and pepper.

Place the chicken breasts in a baking dish. Pour the prepared lemon herb mixture over the chicken, ensuring they are well coated.

Bake the chicken in the preheated oven for about 25-30 minutes or until the chicken is cooked through, and the juices run clear when pierced with a fork.

Roasted Potatoes:

While the chicken is baking, spread the diced potatoes on a baking sheet.

Drizzle olive oil over the potatoes and sprinkle with paprika, dried parsley, salt, and pepper. Toss to coat the potatoes evenly.

Place the baking sheet in the oven and roast the potatoes for about 25-30 minutes or until they are golden brown and crispy on the outside, stirring occasionally for even cooking.

Serving:

Serve the lemon herb chicken alongside the roasted potatoes.

Optionally, garnish the chicken with additional lemon slices or fresh herbs for presentation.

Baked Cod with Herbed Quinoa Pilaf

Ingredients:

For the Baked Cod:

4 cod fillets

2 tablespoons olive oil

2 cloves garlic, minced

Zest and juice of 1 lemon

1 teaspoon dried oregano

1 teaspoon dried thyme

Salt and pepper to taste

Lemon wedges for serving

For the Herbed Quinoa Pilaf:

1 cup quinoa, rinsed

2 cups low-sodium vegetable broth or water

1 tablespoon olive oil

2 cloves garlic, minced

1/4 cup chopped fresh parsley

1/4 cup chopped fresh cilantro

Salt and pepper to taste

Instructions:

Baked Cod:

Preheat your oven to 400°F (200°C).

Place the cod fillets in a baking dish.

In a small bowl, mix together the olive oil, minced garlic, lemon zest, lemon juice, dried oregano, dried thyme, salt, and pepper.

Brush the cod fillets with the prepared mixture, ensuring they are well coated.

Bake the cod in the preheated oven for about 12-15 minutes or until the fish is cooked through and flakes easily with a fork.

Once done, remove the cod from the oven and serve with lemon wedges.

Herbed Quinoa Pilaf:

In a saucepan, combine the rinsed quinoa and low-sodium vegetable broth or water. Bring it to a boil, then reduce heat to low, cover, and simmer for 15-20 minutes or until the liquid is absorbed and the quinoa is cooked.

In a separate pan, heat olive oil over medium heat.

Add minced garlic to the pan and sauté for about 30 seconds until fragrant.

Add the cooked quinoa to the pan with garlic.

Stir in chopped fresh parsley and chopped fresh cilantro.

Season the herbed quinoa pilaf with salt and pepper to taste.

Serving:

Serve the baked cod alongside a portion of herbed quinoa pilaf.

Optionally, garnish with additional fresh herbs before serving.

IBS RELIEF DESSERT RECIPES

Banana-Oat Cookies

Ingredients:

2 ripe bananas, mashed

2 cups old-fashioned oats (certified gluten-free if needed)

1/4 cup chopped walnuts or pecans (optional)

1/4 cup dark chocolate chips (optional)

1 teaspoon ground cinnamon

1 teaspoon vanilla extract

Pinch of salt

Instructions:

Preheat your oven to 350°F (175°C). Line a baking sheet with parchment paper.

In a mixing bowl, combine the mashed bananas, oats, chopped nuts (if using), chocolate chips (if using), ground cinnamon, vanilla extract, and a pinch of salt. Mix until all ingredients are well combined.

Let the mixture sit for about 5-10 minutes to allow the oats to absorb some moisture.

Using a spoon or cookie scoop, drop portions of the mixture onto the prepared baking sheet, shaping them into cookies.

Bake for 12-15 minutes or until the cookies are golden brown around the edges.

Once done, remove the cookies from the oven and let them cool on a wire rack before serving.

Coconut Rice Pudding with Berries

Ingredients:

1 cup Arborio rice (or other short-grain rice)

4 cups low FODMAP lactose-free milk or almond milk

1/4 cup maple syrup or low FODMAP sweetener

1 teaspoon vanilla extract

1/2 cup unsweetened shredded coconut

Mixed berries for topping (e.g., strawberries, blueberries, raspberries)

Instructions:

In a saucepan, combine the rice and lactose-free milk or almond milk. Bring it to a boil over medium heat.

Reduce the heat to low and simmer, stirring occasionally, for about 30-35 minutes or until the rice is cooked and the mixture thickens.

Stir in the maple syrup (or low FODMAP sweetener), vanilla extract, and shredded coconut. Cook for an additional 5 minutes, stirring occasionally.

Remove the saucepan from heat and let the rice pudding cool for a few minutes.

Transfer the rice pudding to individual serving bowls or glasses.

Top the rice pudding with mixed berries.

Optionally, refrigerate the rice pudding before serving to chill it or serve it warm.

Gluten-Free Blueberry Almond Cake

Ingredients:

1 cup almond flour

1/4 cup gluten-free all-purpose flour

1/4 cup cornstarch

1 teaspoon baking powder

1/4 teaspoon salt

1/2 cup unsalted butter, softened

3/4 cup granulated sugar or low FODMAP sweetener

2 large eggs, room temperature

1 teaspoon vanilla extract

1/2 cup lactose-free milk or almond milk

1 cup fresh or frozen blueberries (if using frozen, do not thaw)

Instructions:

Preheat your oven to 350°F (175°C). Grease and line an 8-inch round cake pan with parchment paper.

In a bowl, whisk together the almond flour, gluten-free all-purpose flour, cornstarch, baking powder, and salt. Set aside.

In another bowl, cream together the softened butter and granulated sugar (or low FODMAP sweetener) until light and fluffy.

Add the eggs one at a time, beating well after each addition. Stir in the vanilla extract.

Gradually add the dry flour mixture to the wet ingredients, alternating with the lactose-free milk or almond milk, and mixing until just combined.

Gently fold in the blueberries into the batter.

Pour the batter into the prepared cake pan and spread it evenly.

Bake for 35-40 minutes or until a toothpick inserted into the center comes out clean.

Allow the cake to cool in the pan for 10 minutes before transferring it to a wire rack to cool completely.

Vanilla Chia Pudding with Fresh Fruit

Ingredients:

1/4 cup chia seeds

1 cup lactose-free milk or almond milk

1 tablespoon maple syrup or low FODMAP sweetener

1 teaspoon vanilla extract

Fresh mixed fruit (such as strawberries, kiwi, and pineapple), sliced

Instructions:

In a bowl or jar, mix together the chia seeds, lactose-free milk or almond milk, maple syrup (or low FODMAP sweetener), and vanilla extract.

Stir the mixture well to combine all the ingredients.

Cover the bowl or jar and refrigerate for at least 2-3 hours or overnight to allow the chia seeds to absorb the liquid and thicken, creating a pudding-like consistency.

Once the chia pudding has set, give it a good stir.

Serve the vanilla chia pudding in individual bowls or glasses.

Top the pudding with slices of fresh mixed fruit.

Maple Cinnamon Roasted Almonds

Ingredients:

2 cups whole almonds

2 tablespoons maple syrup (use pure maple syrup for low FODMAP)

1 teaspoon ground cinnamon

1/4 teaspoon salt

Instructions:

Preheat the oven: Preheat your oven to 300°F (150°C). Line a baking sheet with parchment paper.

Prepare the almonds: In a mixing bowl, combine the almonds, maple syrup, ground cinnamon, and salt. Toss until the almonds are evenly coated.

Roast the almonds: Spread the almonds in a single layer on the prepared baking sheet. Roast in the preheated oven for about 20-25 minutes, stirring occasionally to prevent burning. Keep an eye on them in the last few minutes as they can quickly go from toasted to burnt.

Cool and serve: Once the almonds are fragrant and golden brown, remove them from the oven and allow them to cool completely. The maple cinnamon roasted almonds can be stored in an airtight container once cooled.

Berry Chia Seed Pudding

Ingredients:

1 cup unsweetened almond milk (or lactose-free milk)

1/4 cup chia seeds

1 tablespoon maple syrup (use pure maple syrup for low FODMAP)

1/2 teaspoon vanilla extract

1 cup mixed low FODMAP berries (strawberries, blueberries, raspberries)

Instructions:

Prepare the chia pudding: In a bowl or jar, combine the almond milk, chia seeds, maple syrup, and vanilla extract. Stir well to combine. Cover the bowl or jar and refrigerate for at least

4 hours or overnight, allowing the chia seeds to absorb the liquid and form a pudding-like consistency.

Prepare the berries: Wash and slice the mixed berries.

Assemble the pudding: Once the chia seed mixture has thickened into a pudding-like consistency, spoon it into serving bowls or glasses. Top each serving with the mixed berries.

Serve: Serve the Low FODMAP Berry Chia Seed Pudding chilled.

Banana-Oat Cookies

Ingredients:

2 ripe bananas

1 cup rolled oats (ensure they're certified gluten-free if needed)

2 tablespoons unsweetened shredded coconut

2 tablespoons dark chocolate chips (check for no high FODMAP ingredients)

1 tablespoon maple syrup (use pure maple syrup for low FODMAP)

1/2 teaspoon vanilla extract

Pinch of cinnamon (optional)

Instructions:

Preheat the oven: Preheat your oven to 350°F (175°C). Line a baking sheet with parchment paper.

Mash the bananas: In a mixing bowl, mash the ripe bananas with a fork until smooth.

Add the remaining ingredients: Add rolled oats, shredded coconut, dark chocolate chips, maple syrup, vanilla extract, and a pinch of cinnamon (if using) to the mashed bananas. Stir well to combine all the ingredients.

Form cookies: Take spoonfuls of the mixture and place them onto the prepared baking sheet, shaping them into cookie shapes with the back of the spoon.

Bake the cookies: Place the baking sheet in the preheated oven and bake for 12-15 minutes or until the cookies are golden and firm.

Cool and serve: Once done, remove the cookies from the oven and let them cool on a wire rack.

Enjoy these delicious low FODMAP Banana-Oat Cookies as a guilt-free dessert or snack!

Chocolate Avocado Mousse

Ingredients:

2 ripe avocados

1/4 cup unsweetened cocoa powder

1/4 cup maple syrup (use pure maple syrup for low FODMAP)

1 teaspoon vanilla extract

Pinch of salt

Optional toppings: Fresh berries, shredded coconut, or chopped nuts (check for low FODMAP options)

Instructions:

Prepare the avocados: Cut the avocados in half, remove the pits, and scoop the flesh into a food processor or blender.

Blend ingredients: Add cocoa powder, maple syrup, vanilla extract, and a pinch of salt to the avocado in the food processor or blender. Blend until smooth and creamy, scraping down the sides as needed to ensure everything is well combined.

Chill the mousse: Transfer the chocolate avocado mixture to a bowl or individual serving cups. Cover and refrigerate for at least 30 minutes to allow the mousse to chill and set.

Serve: Once chilled, serve the Low FODMAP Chocolate Avocado Mousse topped with fresh berries, shredded coconut, or chopped nuts for added texture and flavor.

Peanut Butter Banana Ice Cream

Ingredients:

4 ripe bananas, peeled, sliced, and frozen

2 tablespoons peanut butter (ensure it's made with just peanuts and salt for low FODMAP)

1-2 tablespoons maple syrup (use pure maple syrup for low FODMAP, adjust sweetness to taste)

1 teaspoon vanilla extract

Instructions:

Freeze the bananas: Slice the ripe bananas into coins and place them in a freezer-safe container. Freeze the banana slices for at least 4 hours or until frozen solid.

Blend ingredients: Once the bananas are frozen, place them in a food processor or blender. Add the peanut butter, maple syrup (start with 1 tablespoon), and vanilla extract.

Blend until creamy: Blend the ingredients until they form a smooth and creamy texture, stopping occasionally to scrape down the sides of the processor or blender. Taste and add more maple syrup if additional sweetness is desired.

Serve immediately: Scoop the Low FODMAP Peanut Butter Banana Ice Cream into bowls and enjoy immediately as soft-serve ice cream or transfer it to a container and freeze for a firmer texture.

Lemon Coconut Energy Balls

Ingredients:

1 cup unsweetened shredded coconut

1/2 cup almond flour

Zest of 1 lemon

Juice of 1/2 lemon

2 tablespoons maple syrup (use pure maple syrup for low FODMAP)

1 tablespoon melted coconut oil

Pinch of salt

Extra shredded coconut for rolling (optional)

Instructions:

Combine ingredients: In a mixing bowl, combine the unsweetened shredded coconut, almond flour, lemon zest, lemon juice, maple syrup, melted coconut oil, and a pinch of salt. Mix well until the ingredients are evenly incorporated.

Form into balls: Using your hands, take small portions of the mixture and roll them into balls. If the mixture is too crumbly to form into balls, add a little more melted coconut oil to help bind it together.

Roll in shredded coconut (optional): If desired, roll the formed balls in additional shredded coconut for an extra coating.

Chill and serve: Place the Lemon Coconut Energy Balls on a plate or tray and refrigerate them for at least 30 minutes to set.

Raspberry Chia Pudding

Ingredients:

1 cup unsweetened almond milk (or lactose-free milk)

1/4 cup chia seeds

1 tablespoon maple syrup (use pure maple syrup for low FODMAP)

1/2 teaspoon vanilla extract

1/2 cup fresh raspberries (or any other low FODMAP berries)

Instructions:

Prepare the chia pudding: In a bowl or jar, mix together the almond milk, chia seeds, maple syrup, and vanilla extract. Stir well until all ingredients are combined. Cover the bowl or jar and refrigerate for at least 2 hours or overnight, allowing the chia seeds to absorb the liquid and thicken into a pudding-like consistency.

Blend the raspberries: In a blender or food processor, puree the fresh raspberries until smooth. If desired, strain the puree through a fine mesh sieve to remove seeds.

Assemble the pudding: Once the chia seed mixture has thickened into a pudding-like consistency, spoon it into serving glasses or bowls. Top the chia pudding with the raspberry puree.

Serve: Serve the Low FODMAP Raspberry Chia Pudding chilled.

Cinnamon Baked Apples

Ingredients:

4 medium-sized firm apples (such as Gala or Fuji)

2 tablespoons maple syrup (use pure maple syrup for low FODMAP)

1 tablespoon melted coconut oil or butter (for lactose-free option)

1 teaspoon ground cinnamon

1/4 teaspoon ground nutmeg (optional)

Chopped nuts (almonds, walnuts) for topping (optional)

Instructions:

Preheat the oven: Preheat your oven to 375°F (190°C).

Prepare the apples: Wash the apples thoroughly and remove the cores, creating a hollow space in the center. You can use an apple corer or a knife to carefully remove the core without cutting through the bottom of the apples.

Mix the filling: In a small bowl, mix together the maple syrup, melted coconut oil or butter, ground cinnamon, and ground nutmeg (if using).

Fill the apples: Place the cored apples on a baking dish or tray. Spoon the cinnamon mixture into each apple, distributing it evenly among them.

Bake the apples: Bake the apples in the preheated oven for about 25-30 minutes or until they are tender and lightly browned.

Serve: Once baked, remove the apples from the oven and let them cool slightly. You can optionally sprinkle chopped nuts on top for added texture.

Chocolate-Dipped Strawberries

Ingredients:

1 pint fresh strawberries, rinsed and dried

4 ounces dark chocolate (check for no high FODMAP ingredients), chopped

1 tablespoon coconut oil

Optional toppings: Crushed nuts (such as almonds or pecans), shredded coconut (unsweetened), or sea salt flakes

Instructions:

Prepare the strawberries: Line a baking sheet or tray with parchment paper. Ensure the strawberries are thoroughly dried after rinsing to allow the chocolate to stick better.

Melt the chocolate: In a microwave-safe bowl or using a double boiler, melt the dark chocolate and coconut oil together in short intervals, stirring frequently until smooth and fully melted.

Dip the strawberries: Holding each strawberry by the stem, dip it into the melted chocolate, swirling to coat about two-thirds of the berry. Allow any excess chocolate to drip off.

Add toppings (optional): If desired, immediately sprinkle the dipped strawberries with crushed nuts, shredded coconut, or a pinch of sea salt flakes before the chocolate sets.

Set and chill: Place the chocolate-dipped strawberries onto the prepared baking sheet. Refrigerate them for about 15-20 minutes or until the chocolate is set.

Serve: Once the chocolate is firm, arrange the Low FODMAP Chocolate-Dipped Strawberries on a plate and serve as a delightful dessert.

Chocolate Banana Smoothie Bowl

Ingredients:

2 ripe bananas, frozen

2 tablespoons unsweetened cocoa powder

1/2 cup lactose-free yogurt or coconut yogurt

1/4 cup almond milk or lactose-free milk

1 tablespoon maple syrup or low FODMAP sweetener (optional)

Toppings: Sliced strawberries, blueberries, shredded coconut, sliced almonds, chia seeds

Instructions:

In a blender, combine the frozen bananas, unsweetened cocoa powder, lactose-free yogurt or coconut yogurt, almond milk (or lactose-free milk), and maple syrup or low FODMAP sweetener (if using).

Blend the ingredients until smooth and creamy. You may need to stop and scrape down the sides of the blender to ensure everything is well mixed.

Pour the chocolate banana smoothie into a bowl.

Top the smoothie bowl with sliced strawberries, blueberries, shredded coconut, sliced almonds, chia seeds, or any other desired toppings.

Lemon Poppy Seed Muffins

Ingredients:

1 1/2 cups gluten-free all-purpose flour

1/2 cup almond flour

1/2 cup granulated sugar or low FODMAP sweetener

2 tablespoons poppy seeds

1 tablespoon baking powder

1/2 teaspoon baking soda

1/4 teaspoon salt

Zest of 2 lemons

1/4 cup lemon juice

1/2 cup lactose-free milk or almond milk

1/3 cup melted coconut oil or vegetable oil

2 eggs

1 teaspoon vanilla extract

Instructions:

Preheat your oven to 350°F (175°C). Line a muffin tin with paper liners or grease the muffin cups.

In a large bowl, whisk together the gluten-free all-purpose flour, almond flour, granulated sugar (or low FODMAP sweetener), poppy seeds, baking powder, baking soda, salt, and lemon zest.

In a separate bowl, mix together the lemon juice, lactose-free milk or almond milk, melted coconut oil or vegetable oil, eggs, and vanilla extract.

Pour the wet ingredients into the dry ingredients and gently fold them together until just combined. Do not overmix.

Spoon the batter into the prepared muffin cups, filling them about 3/4 full.

Bake for 18-20 minutes or until a toothpick inserted into the center of a muffin comes out clean.

Allow the muffins to cool in the pan for a few minutes before transferring them to a wire rack to cool completely.

Almond Butter and Banana Rice Cakes

Ingredients:

Rice cakes (gluten-free, if needed)

Almond butter (unsweetened)

Ripe bananas, thinly sliced

Cinnamon (optional)

Honey or maple syrup (optional, for added sweetness)

Instructions:

Spread a generous layer of almond butter onto each rice cake.

Top the almond butter with thinly sliced ripe bananas, arranging them evenly over the rice cake.

Optionally, sprinkle a pinch of cinnamon over the bananas for added flavor.

If desired, drizzle a small amount of honey or maple syrup over the bananas for extra sweetness.

Serve immediately.

IBS RELIEF SOUP RECIPES

PUMPKIN NOODLE SOUP

INGREDIENTS

2 tbsp tandoori spices (make sure no low FODMAP ingredients have been added. The mix that I used contained: paprika, cilantro, salt, cumin, pepper, ginger, chilli, cinnamon and laurel)

1/2 tbsp fresh ginger

1/2 tsp turmeric

1/2 tsp ground cloves

1/4 tsp cayenne pepper

A small handful of fresh cilantro

A splash of lemon juice

One stalk of spring onion

FOR THE SOUP

200 ml (6.7 oz) coconut milk

750 ml (3.2 cups) stock (use a low FODMAP stock cube)

400 g (14.1) oz pumpkin in cubes

1 tsp fish sauce (leave this out to make the recipe vegan)

150 g (5.3 oz) oyster mushrooms

1 tbsp brown sugar

150 g (5.3 oz) gluten-free noodles

Fresh basil

Unsalted peanuts

Cook Mode Prevent your screen from going dark

INSTRUCTIONS

This recipe is based on this recipe by My Food Story

Cut the ginger, cilantro and spring onion into very small pieces. Put those together with all the spices and a splash of lemon juice in a bowl. Make this into a paste using a hand blender.

Boil the pumpkin cubes in a pan with boiling water for 10 minutes. Drain them well and use a hand mixer to make a pumpkin puree.

Heat some oil in a soup pan and add the spice paste. Fry this for two minutes while you stir now and then. Add the pumpkin puree, fish sauce and 600 ml stock.

Scrub the oyster mushrooms clean, cut them into pieces and add them together with the sugar and a pinch of salt to the soup.

Bring the soup to a boil and leave to boil for about 10 minutes.

Boil the noodles according to the instruction on the package. Drain them and rinse them with cold water, so they don't stick.

Add, after 10 minutes of cooking, the rest of the stock and the coconut milk. Leave the soup to boil for another 5 minutes.

Add some fresh basil and the noodles to the soup and stir together. Turn off the heat and leave the soup to rest for 5 minutes with the lid on the pan.

Serve the soup with some extra basil and chopped peanuts.

BROCCOLI SOUP WITH SAUSAGE

INGREDIENTS

1.5 liter (6 cups) stock (use a low FODMAP stock)

400 g (2.5 cups) celeriac

2 leeks, only the green part

1 large carrot (about 2 cups)

200 g (1 1/8 cups) broccoli heads

2 bay leaves

1 low FODMAP smoked sausage*

Optional: the green of 3 stalks of spring onion

Optional: pieces of baked bacon

Cook Mode Prevent your screen from going dark

INSTRUCTIONS

Peel the celeriac and cut into cubes. Shop the green part of the leeks. Cut the carrot into cubes and the broccoli into florets.

Put all vegetables, the celeriac and the bay leaves in a pan and pour the stock on top.

Leave to boil until the vegetables are soft (about 15 minutes) and remove the bay leaves. Blend the soup with an immersion blender until smooth. Season with pepper and salt.

Cut the smoked sausage into pieces and add to the soup. Leave the soup to simmer for half an hour on low heat.

If you want to add bacon: bake it in a separate pan and add to the soup when you serve it.

Butternut Squash Soup

Ingredients:

1 medium butternut squash, peeled, seeded, and cubed

1 tablespoon olive oil

1 onion, chopped

2 carrots, chopped

2 celery stalks, chopped

3 cloves garlic, minced

4 cups low-sodium vegetable broth

1 teaspoon ground cumin

1/2 teaspoon ground cinnamon

Salt and pepper to taste

Coconut milk or lactose-free cream for garnish (optional)

Fresh parsley or chives for garnish (optional)

Instructions:

In a large pot, heat the olive oil over medium heat.

Add the chopped onion, carrots, and celery. Sauté for about 5-7 minutes until they begin to soften.

Add the minced garlic and cook for an additional minute until fragrant.

Stir in the cubed butternut squash, ground cumin, ground cinnamon, salt, and pepper.

Cook for another 5 minutes, stirring occasionally.

Pour in the low-sodium vegetable broth. Bring the mixture to a boil, then reduce the heat to low. Cover the pot and simmer for 20-25 minutes or until the butternut squash is tender.

Remove the pot from heat and let the soup cool slightly.

Using an immersion blender or regular blender, carefully blend the soup until smooth and creamy.

Return the soup to the pot and reheat if necessary.

Serve the butternut squash soup hot, garnished with a drizzle of coconut milk or lactose-free cream and fresh parsley or chives if desired.

Carrot and Ginger Soup

Ingredients:

1 tablespoon olive oil

1 pound carrots, peeled and chopped

1 potato, peeled and diced

1-inch piece of ginger, peeled and minced

4 cups low-sodium vegetable broth

Salt and pepper to taste

Fresh chives for garnish (optional)

Instructions:

Heat olive oil in a large pot over medium heat.

Add chopped carrots, diced potato, and minced ginger to the pot. Sauté for about 5 minutes, stirring occasionally.

Pour in the low-sodium vegetable broth, bring the mixture to a boil, then reduce the heat to low. Cover the pot and let it simmer for about 20-25 minutes or until the vegetables are tender.

Remove the pot from heat and let the mixture cool slightly.

Using an immersion blender or regular blender, carefully blend the soup until smooth.

Return the soup to the pot and reheat if necessary.

Season the soup with salt and pepper to taste.

Serve the carrot and ginger soup hot, garnished with fresh chives if desired.

Chicken and Vegetable Soup

Ingredients:

1 tablespoon olive oil

1 pound boneless, skinless chicken breasts, diced

1 onion, chopped

2 carrots, diced

2 celery stalks, diced

3 cloves garlic, minced

6 cups low-sodium chicken broth

1 teaspoon dried thyme

1 teaspoon dried oregano

Salt and pepper to taste

2 cups baby spinach or kale, chopped

Fresh parsley for garnish (optional)

Instructions:

In a large pot, heat the olive oil over medium heat.

Add the diced chicken and cook until it's no longer pink. Remove the chicken from the pot and set it aside.

In the same pot, add the chopped onion, diced carrots, and diced celery. Sauté for about 5 minutes until they start to soften.

Add the minced garlic and cook for an additional minute until fragrant.

Pour in the low-sodium chicken broth and bring it to a boil.

Add the dried thyme, dried oregano, salt, and pepper. Stir well.

Reduce the heat to low and simmer the soup for about 15-20 minutes.

Add the cooked chicken back into the pot and simmer for an additional 5 minutes.

Stir in the chopped baby spinach or kale and cook until wilted.

Taste and adjust the seasoning if needed.

Serve the chicken and vegetable soup hot, garnished with fresh parsley if desired.

Lentil Soup

Ingredients:

1 cup dried lentils, rinsed and drained

1 tablespoon olive oil

1 onion, chopped

2 carrots, diced

2 celery stalks, diced

3 cloves garlic, minced

6 cups low-sodium vegetable broth

1 teaspoon ground cumin

1 teaspoon ground coriander

1/2 teaspoon smoked paprika

Salt and pepper to taste

2 tablespoons fresh lemon juice

Fresh parsley for garnish (optional)

Instructions:

In a large pot, heat the olive oil over medium heat.

Add the chopped onion, diced carrots, and diced celery. Sauté for about 5 minutes until they start to soften.

Add the minced garlic and cook for an additional minute until fragrant.

Pour in the low-sodium vegetable broth and add the rinsed lentils.

Stir in the ground cumin, ground coriander, smoked paprika, salt, and pepper. Mix well.

Bring the soup to a boil, then reduce the heat to low. Cover the pot and let it simmer for about 25-30 minutes or until the lentils are tender.

Once the lentils are cooked, stir in the fresh lemon juice.

Taste and adjust the seasoning if needed.

Serve the lentil soup hot, garnished with fresh parsley if desired.

Lemon Sorbet

Ingredients:

1 cup water

1/2 cup pure maple syrup (for a sweeter sorbet, adjust the quantity as desired)

Zest of 2 lemons

1 cup freshly squeezed lemon juice (from about
4-6 lemons)

Instructions:

Prepare the syrup: In a saucepan, combine
water and maple syrup. Bring the mixture to a
gentle boil, stirring occasionally. Once boiling,
remove it from heat and let it cool to room
temperature.

Prepare the lemon mixture: In a bowl, combine
the lemon zest and freshly squeezed lemon
juice.

Combine the mixtures: Once the syrup has cooled, mix it with the lemon juice and zest mixture. Stir well to combine.

Chill and churn: Pour the mixture into an ice cream maker and churn according to the manufacturer's instructions until it reaches a sorbet-like consistency.

Freeze: Transfer the churned sorbet into a freezer-safe container. Cover it and freeze for at least 4-6 hours or until it's firm enough to scoop.

Serve: Scoop the Low FODMAP Lemon Sorbet into serving bowls or cones. Enjoy this refreshing and tangy treat!

Tomato Basil Soup

Ingredients:

2 tablespoons olive oil

1 cup carrots, diced

1 cup celery, diced

2 cups canned crushed tomatoes (check for no high FODMAP ingredients)

4 cups low FODMAP vegetable broth

1 teaspoon dried basil

Salt and pepper to taste

Fresh basil leaves for garnish (optional)

Instructions:

Saute vegetables: In a large pot, heat olive oil over medium heat. Add diced carrots and celery. Saute for about 5-7 minutes until the vegetables soften.

Add tomatoes and broth: Pour in the canned crushed tomatoes and low FODMAP vegetable broth. Stir well to combine.

Season and simmer: Add the dried basil, salt, and pepper. Bring the mixture to a simmer. Reduce the heat and let it simmer uncovered for 15-20 minutes, allowing the flavors to meld.

Blend (optional): For a smoother texture, use an immersion blender or transfer the soup in batches to a blender and blend until smooth.

Serve: Ladle the Low FODMAP Tomato Basil Soup into bowls. Garnish with fresh basil leaves if desired and serve warm.

Butternut Squash Soup

Ingredients:

1 medium butternut squash, peeled, seeded, and diced (about 4 cups)

1 tablespoon olive oil

1 cup carrots, diced

1 cup potatoes, peeled and diced

4 cups low FODMAP vegetable broth

1 teaspoon ground cumin

1/2 teaspoon ground cinnamon

Salt and pepper to taste

Fresh chives (green parts only) for garnish (optional)

Instructions:

Roast the squash: Preheat your oven to 400°F (200°C). Place the diced butternut squash on a baking sheet, drizzle with olive oil, and season lightly with salt. Roast for about 25-30 minutes or until the squash is tender and slightly caramelized. Remove from the oven and set aside.

Saute vegetables: In a large pot, heat olive oil over medium heat. Add diced carrots and potatoes. Saute for about 5-7 minutes until they begin to soften.

Add roasted squash and broth: Add the roasted butternut squash to the pot along with the low FODMAP vegetable broth. Stir well.

Season and simmer: Stir in the ground cumin, ground cinnamon, salt, and pepper. Bring the mixture to a boil, then reduce the heat and let it simmer for 15-20 minutes, allowing the flavors to meld.

Blend (optional): Use an immersion blender or transfer the soup in batches to a blender and blend until smooth.

Serve: Ladle the Low FODMAP Butternut Squash Soup into bowls. Garnish with fresh chives if desired and serve warm.

Spinach and Potato Soup

Ingredients:

1 tablespoon olive oil

2 cups potatoes, peeled and diced

1 cup carrots, diced

1 cup spinach, chopped

4 cups low FODMAP vegetable broth

1 teaspoon dried thyme

Salt and pepper to taste

Fresh parsley for garnish (optional)

Instructions:

Saute vegetables: In a large pot, heat olive oil over medium heat. Add diced potatoes and carrots. Saute for about 5-7 minutes until they start to soften.

Add broth and simmer: Pour in the low FODMAP vegetable broth and chopped spinach. Stir well. Add dried thyme, salt, and pepper. Bring the mixture to a boil, then reduce the heat and let it simmer for 15-20 minutes or until the vegetables are tender.

Blend (optional): For a smoother consistency, use an immersion blender or transfer a portion of the soup to a blender and blend until desired smoothness. Return it to the pot and mix well.

Serve: Ladle the Low FODMAP Spinach and Potato Soup into bowls. Garnish with fresh parsley if desired and serve warm.

Lentil and Vegetable Soup

Ingredients:

1 tablespoon olive oil

1 cup carrots, diced

1 cup zucchini, diced

1 cup bell peppers (red or yellow), diced

1 cup diced tomatoes (canned or fresh)

1 cup dry lentils, rinsed and drained

6 cups low FODMAP vegetable broth

1 teaspoon dried thyme

1 teaspoon ground cumin

Salt and pepper to taste

Fresh parsley for garnish (optional)

Instructions:

Saute vegetables: In a large pot, heat olive oil
over medium heat. Add diced carrots, zucchini,

and bell peppers. Saute for about 5 minutes until they start to soften.

Add lentils and broth: Add diced tomatoes, rinsed lentils, low FODMAP vegetable broth, dried thyme, and ground cumin to the pot. Stir well.

Simmer: Bring the mixture to a boil, then reduce the heat to a simmer. Cover and let it cook for about 25-30 minutes or until the lentils and vegetables are tender.

Season: Season the soup with salt and pepper to taste.

Serve: Ladle the Low FODMAP Lentil and Vegetable Soup into bowls. Garnish with fresh parsley if desired and serve hot.

Broccoli and Potato Soup

Ingredients:

1 tablespoon olive oil

2 cups broccoli florets

2 cups potatoes, peeled and diced

1 cup carrots, diced

4 cups low FODMAP vegetable broth

1 teaspoon dried thyme

Salt and pepper to taste

Fresh chives (green parts only) for garnish (optional)

Instructions:

Saute vegetables: In a large pot, heat olive oil over medium heat. Add diced potatoes and carrots. Saute for about 5 minutes until they start to soften.

Add broth and broccoli: Pour in the low FODMAP vegetable broth. Add broccoli florets and dried thyme. Stir well.

Simmer: Bring the mixture to a boil, then reduce the heat to a simmer. Cover and let it cook for about 15-20 minutes or until the vegetables are tender.

Blend (optional): For a creamier texture, use an immersion blender or transfer a portion of the soup to a blender and blend until desired consistency. Return it to the pot and mix well.

Season: Season the soup with salt and pepper to taste.

Serve: Ladle the Low FODMAP Broccoli and Potato Soup into bowls. Garnish with fresh chives if desired and serve warm.

Spiced Pumpkin Soup

Ingredients:

1 tablespoon olive oil

1 cup canned pumpkin puree (ensure no high FODMAP ingredients)

2 cups carrots, peeled and chopped

1 cup parsnips, peeled and chopped

4 cups low FODMAP vegetable broth

1 teaspoon ground cumin

1/2 teaspoon ground ginger

1/4 teaspoon ground nutmeg

Salt and pepper to taste

Fresh parsley for garnish (optional)

Instructions:

Saute vegetables: In a large pot, heat olive oil over medium heat. Add chopped carrots and parsnips. Saute for about 5-7 minutes until they start to soften.

Add pumpkin and broth: Stir in the canned pumpkin puree, low FODMAP vegetable broth, ground cumin, ground ginger, and ground nutmeg. Mix well.

Simmer: Bring the mixture to a boil, then reduce the heat to a simmer. Cover and let it cook for about 20-25 minutes or until the vegetables are tender.

Blend (optional): For a smoother texture, use an immersion blender or transfer a portion of the soup to a blender and blend until desired consistency. Return it to the pot and mix well.

Season: Season the soup with salt and pepper to taste.

Serve: Ladle the Low FODMAP Spiced Pumpkin Soup into bowls. Garnish with fresh parsley if desired and serve warm.

Roasted Red Pepper Soup

Ingredients:

4 red bell peppers

1 tablespoon olive oil

1 cup carrots, diced

1 cup potatoes, diced

4 cups low FODMAP vegetable broth

1 teaspoon dried basil

1/2 teaspoon smoked paprika

Salt and pepper to taste

Fresh basil leaves for garnish (optional)

Instructions:

Roast the bell peppers: Preheat the oven to 400°F (200°C). Place the whole red bell peppers on a baking sheet and roast them in the oven for about 25-30 minutes, turning occasionally, until the skin is charred and blistered. Remove from the oven and let them cool. Once cooled, peel off the skin, remove seeds, and chop the roasted peppers.

Saute vegetables: In a large pot, heat olive oil over medium heat. Add diced carrots and potatoes. Saute for about 5 minutes until they start to soften.

Add broth and roasted peppers: Pour in the low FODMAP vegetable broth and add the chopped roasted red peppers. Stir well.

Season and simmer: Add dried basil, smoked paprika, salt, and pepper. Bring the mixture to a boil, then reduce the heat to a simmer. Cover and let it cook for about 15-20 minutes or until the vegetables are tender.

Blend (optional): For a smoother texture, use an immersion blender or transfer a portion of the soup to a blender and blend until desired consistency. Return it to the pot and mix well.

Serve: Ladle the Low FODMAP Roasted Red Pepper Soup into bowls. Garnish with fresh basil leaves if desired and serve warm.

Lemon Chicken Soup

Ingredients:

1 tablespoon olive oil

2 boneless, skinless chicken breasts, diced

1 cup carrots, diced

1 cup celery, diced

6 cups low FODMAP chicken broth

Zest and juice of 1 lemon

1 teaspoon dried thyme

Salt and pepper to taste

Fresh parsley for garnish (optional)

Instructions:

Saute chicken and vegetables: In a large pot, heat olive oil over medium heat. Add diced chicken breasts and cook until lightly browned. Add diced carrots and celery. Saute for about 5 minutes until the vegetables begin to soften.

Add broth and seasonings: Pour in the low FODMAP chicken broth. Add the lemon zest, lemon juice, dried thyme, salt, and pepper. Stir well.

Simmer: Bring the mixture to a boil, then reduce the heat to a simmer. Cover and let it cook for about 15-20 minutes or until the chicken is cooked through and the vegetables are tender.

Serve: Ladle the Low FODMAP Lemon Chicken Soup into bowls. Garnish with fresh parsley if desired and serve hot.